COMMUNITY INVOLVEMENT IN HEALTH

(Short loan)
Community Involvement in Health
From Passive Recipients to Active Participants

Jan Smithies and Georgina Webster
Labyrinth Training and Consultancy

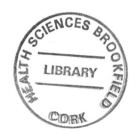

ASHGATE

Published by
Ashgate Publishing Limited
Gower House
Croft Road
Aldershot
Hants GU11 3HR
England

Ashgate Publishing Company
Suite 420
101 Cherry Street
Burlington, VT 05401-4405
USA

Ashgate website: http://www.ashgate.com

Reprinted 2001, 2004

British Library Cataloguing in Publication Data
Smithies, Jan
   Community involvement in health : from passive recipients
   to active participants
   1. Community health services – Great Britain 2. Community
   health services – Great Britain – Citizen participation
   I. Title II. Webster, Georgina
   362.1'2'0941

Library of Congress Cataloging-in-Publication Data
Smithies, Jan.
   Community involvement in health : from passive recipients to
   active participants / Jan Smithies and Georgina Webster.
         p. cm.
      Includes bibliographical references.
      ISBN 1-85742-428-X (hbk).
      1. Community health services—Great Britain—Citizen
   participation. 2. Public health advisory groups—Great Britain.
   3. Medical policy—Great Britain—Citizen participation.
   I. Webster, Georgina. II. Title.
   RA485.S59   1998
   362.1'2'0941—dc21   98-12737
                                              CIP

ISBN 1 85742 428 X

Printed in Great Britain by Biddles Limited, King's Lynn.

Contents

List of figures, tables and boxes

Figures

Tables

Boxes .

List of case studies

Preface

This book brings together both the history of community involvement in health, and ideas and proposals for further developing the potential of this approach. It explores the 'roots' and 'branches' of community involvement in health, drawing together different strands from within and outside the National Health Service, and in particular focusing on communities themselves.

Much innovative and creative work has been undertaken under the broad concept of 'community involvement'. The book comprehensively documents the development of a 'community health movement' in the United Kingdom; it also explores the impact of the rapid changes in the National Health Service on local communities, patients and service users, and ways in which current policy can enhance and enable the general public to be more involved in their own health and well-being and in effective service provision.

Fundamentally the book is concerned with helping to support good practice in relation to community involvement. To this end, models, ideas and case studies are used to illustrate practical ways that people and organisations can enhance their own skills and knowledge. However, we believe that these need to be explored within the wider context of both historical and current policy and theory.

The book advocates that community involvement is an important way forward in building partnerships between local people, health planners, policy makers and providers and wider social welfare agencies. It argues that initiatives which enable people to move from the role of 'passive recipients to active participants' are important if we are to see improvements both in people's health and well-being and in the quality and effectiveness of services which deal with ill health. Involvement needs to be a key feature of a primary health care led NHS.

By raising the profile of community involvement in health we intend that the book will help readers to build up effective practice, and to make clear and effective arguments for why this way of working should be adopted by their own organisation. The contents will be of interest to a wide range of people including health professionals, provider organisations, managers and service planners, purchasers/commissioners, board members, local authority staff, officers and members, community workers and indeed local people who are active in their own communities around health issues. As both theory and practice are explored, the book will be useful to those with substantial experience in this field, as well as to those wishing to learn more as a way of beginning such work. By recording the history and exploring the links between policy and practice the book also has something to offer academic and professional teaching audiences.

Addresses for many of the projects and organisations mentioned in the book are given in the Appendix.

Introduction

This book is divided into three main parts. The first part explores the wider context within which community involvement in health is placed. To this end there are chapters exploring the history of both community involvement in general, and specifically community involvement within health. Although the book is mostly concerned with the United Kingdom, there is also a brief look at the international context. This is then brought up to date in subsequent chapters which bring together a comprehensive overview of what the current situation looks like in terms of policies and practice. Finally, the first part explores why community involvement is important and looks at the benefits to a range of stakeholders, including local people, communities, the NHS, wider social welfare organisations and society as a whole.

The second part is very practical and uses tools, models, approaches, ideas and case studies to help people think about their own practice both within their own organisations and in direct work with local people and communities. We believe that effective community involvement requires skills at a range of levels and across a range of disciplines. We therefore devote space to organisation development and strategic approaches as well as community work skills and techniques. Language and terminology are also explored in some depth here.

Part III contains chapters which explore what needs to change in organisations, in professional training and skills and in communities if the potential of community involvement in health is to be fully realised. Checklists for action and contacts for useful organisations are included here. It finishes with our conclusions and ideas for the future.

It is possible to use the book in several different ways. It can be read through in its entirety. It is also meant to be a reference book which can be returned to and used selectively, perhaps when seeking case studies of good practice, ideas for starting new work, or when in search of ideas about methodologies and practical models, for example.

We have been very active in this field of work for many years. We have extensive experience of working directly with community groups and local people on health and wider social welfare issues, but have also been responsible for the development of policy, professional training and strategic level initiatives at local, district and national levels. We also have some international experience in this field. For the last eight years we have worked as independent consultants and trainers and have pioneered new models, good practice and the furtherment of theory. This book is therefore written from the perspective of experience and from enthusiasm and commitment to community involvement.

We have noted the growth of work aimed at promoting community involvement in health, accelerated by the NHS purchaser/provider split and by specific initiatives such as *Local Voices* (which was issued to all health purchasing organisations by the then National Health Service Management Executive in 1992). Many of those coming into this area of work, both at community and strategic levels, are not aware of the history of work on community involvement in health and do not have access to the wide range of good practice and approaches and models that have been, and are being, developed. This book is therefore an important landmark in logging how far things have come in the UK and an advocate for where things might go in the future.

By using checklists, questions and models at key points in the text we offer the reader the opportunity to engage with the written word and ideas from the point of view of their own practice, philosophy and plans. We are unashamedly enthusiastic about, and committed to, the subject matter, but also seek to explore where policy, practice and theory could be more effectively reconciled.

Part I

Context: the roots and branches of community involvement in health

The current upsurge of interest in developing community involvement in health is fed by two main strands – central government policy with a new focus on the obligations of health and local authorities to listen to, act on the views of, and continuously engage with, their local populations; and a continuous history of community-led action, involving campaigns for a greater say in decisions affecting health and well-being as well as the development of self-help activities. In other words, both 'top down' and 'bottom up' initiatives combine in shaping the direction of community involvement in health today.

Both strands need to be understood to appreciate why community involvement in health in the UK at the present time looks as it does, where its particular dilemmas come from, and how work to promote greater community involvement can most successfully take place.

Part I of the book explores these strands in detail.

1   History: the early roots

Summary

This chapter describes some of the strands of community action that have fed into the development of community involvement in health. It begins by looking briefly at the history of community development within the UK in the twentieth century and the emergence of an organised community development movement from the late 1960s onwards. The next sections describe some of the social movements which have played a crucial role in bringing about community involvement in health, such as feminism, black community action, disability rights, environmental movements and so on. The role of 'radical health professionals' in defining a 'new' public health is also explored. This leads on to describing the positive effect of the 'Health For All' initiative of the World Health Organization and its interpretation internationally, in mobilising community action around health within the UK. The final section highlights the development of health-orientated self-help and lobbying/campaigning groups and organisations as key players in taking forward and shaping community involvement in health.

Community development

Community development began as a recognisable activity within the UK in late Victorian times and many of the attitudes then embodied in it have persisted to modern times. It developed out of the work of a number of charitable organisations such as the Charity Organisation Society, as well as philanthropic bodies and university settlements, as a way of improving the lot of 'the poor' and of dealing with social unrest (Craig 1989). It was, essentially, a paternalistic approach to working with poor people. This approach was reinforced during the 1930s and after through the influence of British colonial experience, particularly in West Africa. Local British administrators were involved in a form of intervention the Colonial Office was to name in 1941 as 'community development'. Communities were encouraged to undertake self-help projects without outside funding in order to improve community facilities and well-being (Hanmer 1991).

However, by the end of the 1940s, community development was also seen as giving a more pro-active role to communities in bringing about change, and the definition of community development offered by the United Nations in 1948 was: 'A movement to promote better living for the whole community, with active participation and if possible on the initiative of the community, but if this initiative is not forthcoming, by the use of techniques for arousing and stimulating it...' (Craig 1989, p. 5).

This definition is still relevant to community development as it is practised today, although the language has changed: we would talk now about 'enabling' rather than 'arousing and stimulating'. These 'techniques' later developed into the skills and tools embodied within community work training and practice. A key concept underlying the use of community work techniques was the notion of 'non-directive' methods of community work practice, developed by T.R Batten, an influential British community work theorist writing in the 1940s and 1950s. His description of this method was based heavily on the colonial experience:

> Workers who adopt this [non-directive] approach no longer try to guide or persuade. They stimulate people to think about their needs, feed in information about possible ways of meeting them, and encourage them to decide for themselves what they will do to meet them. The theory underlying this approach is that people are far more likely to act on what they themselves have freely decided to do than on what a worker has tried to convince them they ought to do. [Craig 1989, p. 5]

Following the end of the Second World War, the development of community work was heavily influenced by the appearance of the Welfare State and of post-war concerns about the 'decline of the community', apparently due to ever-increasing urbanisation and industrialisation. Within this scenario, the role of community development was to re-establish 'community spirit'.[1] At this time most community workers were funded by charitable bodies and employed within new housing developments and community centres, to enable and build a sense of community through self-help community activity. This role was given greater prominence by the British government at the end of the 1960s with the introduction of a number of initiatives designed to tackle social unrest among 'disadvantaged' communities.

The 1960s saw a growing government debate about the problems of what came to be called 'inner city areas'. The debate included discussion of the 'poverty trap', the increase in 'juvenile delinquency' and the existence of 'racial disharmony'. Part of the government response involved the development of a range of similar initiatives designed to address the problems of these areas at community level. These included the setting up of a number of Community Development Projects throughout England and Wales by the Home Office, as joint initiatives with local government, as a way of reaching communities not participating in council services; the creation of new generic Social Services Departments which employed community workers as a strategy for preventative social work; the establishment of local Community Relations Councils employing Community Development Workers, as part of the 1968 Race Relations Act; the Government Urban Aid Programme which financed innovatory projects in inner-city areas, many of which involved the appointment of community workers; the designation of Educational Priority Areas with community education programmes reaching out to local communities, and so on. These initiatives represented a significant increase in government-sponsored community development and a significant growth in community work activities.

This growth in community development in the late 1960s has been sustained to the present day, represented both by a growth in the number of community workers (employed in statutory and voluntary agencies) and a growth in local and national policies and practices designed to support community development work locally. As a result a number of bodies have been established by workers in the field to support and promote community development. These bodies have in common an explicit desire to widen access to community development skills and expertise, and to promote its practice from a 'bottom up' perspective, without confining the practice of community work to a professional elite.

The Association of Community Workers was set up by practitioners in the early 1970s to stimulate co-operation and become a voice for community work. This was followed a decade later by the establishment of the Federation of Community Work Training Groups, again by workers in the field, to stimulate community work training and enable access to such training by local community activists. This in turn helped to establish the Standing Conference on Community Development as a membership organisation aimed at providing an 'umbrella' for all those active and interested in community development, locally and nationally (SCCD et al. 1995). The two latter organisations are funded by central government, initially through the Home Office, briefly through the Department for National Heritage, and latterly again through the Home Office. At the same time Community Matters has developed as a national organisation of locally based community organisations, and as a voice for those active in community development in, usually, an unpaid and voluntary capacity.

Central government also funds voluntary organisations whose remit includes community development, notably the Community Development Foundation. These organisations are different from those listed above in so far as they do not directly represent the 'field' of community work but work to support its activities.

In the thirty years following the 1960s growth, both local and central government have continued to play a major role in funding and shaping community work, community development and community participation. Thus in the UK we now have an experienced community development sector, with a sophisticated and accessible set of skills, knowledge and theory which is available to and has been used by the community health movement to influence the growth of community involvement in health. So far we have, on the whole, concentrated on describing some of the 'top down' influences which have shaped community development in the UK. The next section outlines some of the social movements which have exerted an equally strong influence, from a 'bottom up' perspective.

The influence of social movements

From its beginnings community development has been shaped as much by the activities and energies of communities themselves as by government or philanthropic intervention. For instance, in the early years of this century many working-class movements were as concerned with improving community life in the broadest sense, and organising to do so, as with efforts to improve pay and working conditions (which of course also impact on community life). Examples include the Co-operative Women's Guild which was established in 1883 and campaigned vigorously for the neglected needs of married working women and were successful in organising for state benefits and better health facilities for working mothers (Llewelyn Davies 1977). As autonomous groups, women within the Guild not only campaigned vigorously for maternity rights, women's suffrage, miners' rights and so on, but also established an extensive education programme to help members organise their own groups as well as playing a greater role in public life (Salt et al. 1983). At the same time, the rapidly developing trade union movement and early labour movement, organised autonomously to improve the lot of their members. Health was seen as an important issue in this connection as local working people were encouraged to act as Poor Law Guardians, or as members of Public Health Committees and so on (Mitchell 1977, Liddington 1984). Sometimes their activity was supported by sympathetic outsiders. For instance, one university settlement in the East End of London was actively involved in supporting strikes and encouraging trade union organisation among low-paid workers and dock labourers (Craig 1989).

Again it was the late 1960s which saw a mushrooming of the social movements which exerted an influence on the direction of community work. At this time the notion that the 'community' was something homogenous, or something that ought to be homogenous, was dramatically challenged by the activities of these social movements, such as the civil rights movement, Black Power, Women's Liberation, the student movement, Anarchism and the New Left. They were to be followed shortly by community-based groupings such as the squatters' collectives and Claimants' Unions. These movements largely affected community development through the experiences and ideologies of individual community workers who had been involved in them. They brought the notion of oppression, by class, race or gender, into the work, and the role of the community worker came to be seen by some as helping oppressed groups organise for change.

People involved in these different social movements brought a new energy into the practice of community development, whether they were paid community workers or unpaid volunteers/activists. They also brought new ways of organising. For example, they challenged the notion that the community worker should always be seen as 'non-directive' – was this relevant if the worker saw themselves as a member of an oppressed group or community pressing for change? This was especially significant where community development workers were increasingly being recruited from the communities they were intended to work with. In addition they brought new issues into the community development arena, and new ways of tackling them. Women community workers insisted that health was an important community work issue and should not be left to the health professionals. They also encouraged groups to work in collective and collaborative ways, sharing tasks and roles, instead of following the more traditional and hierarchical way of organising through a committee structure (Hanmer 1991).

Health was explicitly seen as a central issue by many of these movements. Women's organising on health was an early feature of the Women's Liberation Movement, focusing initially on women's reproductive health. 'Gaining control over our bodies' was interpreted partly as a need to create and disseminate accurate information on how the body worked and how it could be affected, as well as a recognition of the need to raise awareness of the social causes of ill health (Hanmer 1991). The Women's Reproductive Rights and Information Centre was set up by health workers in the field to help meet this need.

Equally, health has been a concern of black groups – for instance, the Black Patients and Health Workers Group was set up in the 1970s to express and act on this concern, and the Sickle Cell Society was established in London in 1979 by concerned and active black health professionals and community members (Ogunsola 1991, Douglas 1991). Chapter 2 discusses the role of black community health projects and workers in the emerging community health movement in the UK in more detail. However, it is worth noting here that the funding of black health initiatives by different sections of the NHS, both locally and nationally, has been heavily influenced by the activities and representation of Black Community Health Projects (Douglas 1991, Coke 1991).

More recently the disability rights movement, environmental movements and user and advocacy movements have all played a role in influencing the direction of community involvement in health. In different ways they have all been active in ensuring that the voices of their members do not go unheard. At the same time they have brought their unique perspectives and their practical ways of organising into the community development arena. For instance, People First and other groups of people with learning disabilities have probably played a greater role in the creation of 'jargon-free' ways of communication between organisations and the public than most other groups, and to the benefit of all groups. In this connection, it has been said that the advocacy and user movements have been successful in reaching and enabling the participation of groups in community life which have not been reached by traditional community development groups and organisations (Labyrinth 1994b). The section 'Regeneration initiatives' in Chapter 3 describes the role of the advocacy and user movements in greater detail.

The new public health

Interventions to improve 'public health' originate in the Victorian concern to do something about the uncontrolled spread of infectious diseases which seemed to accompany rapid industrialisation and urbanisation in the early nineteenth century. Edwin Chadwick and his like-minded contemporaries (he was Secretary to the Poor Law Commission established in 1834 and a Commissioner in the General Board of Health established in 1848) saw themselves as key advocates of the importance of public health intervention. Their activities led to the establishment of the public health profession; however, by the beginning of the following century, lay involvement in this profession's work and activities had been discouraged (Webster 1993, p. 3).

However, lay participation in public health has never been entirely destroyed and this has been represented since the 1980s through the rise of the 'New Public Health'. This is a movement of public health professionals and others who have sought to re-emphasise the crucial role that social and environmental factors play in affecting the public's health; and therefore the importance of building alliances between the public and the public health profession in taking action to influence these factors. In this respect the Black report of 1980 and Margaret Whitehead's 'Health Divide', 1987 (Townsend et al. 1992) have been instrumental in highlighting class and regional inequalities in health (Webster 1993, p. 3). Later chapters describe some of the current writings on inequalities in health, but the two reports mentioned here were influential in the creation and maintenance of the New Public Health. This movement set up its own organisation, the Public Health Alliance, in 1989 as an independent voluntary organisation bringing together individuals and organisations committed to public health (PHA 1989).[2]

The emphasis on a social definition of health, and on the importance of lay involvement in public health (which was emphasised by the New Public Health) received international recognition with the development of the World Health Organization strategy of 'Health For All by the Year 2000'.

Health For All

'Health For All by the Year 2000' (HFA 2000) is a World Health Organization-sponsored initiative to which the UK government, as well as other governments world-wide, have signed up and subscribed. It has three basic and overarching aims and principles: community participation, redressing inequalities and intersectoral collaboration (what we would now call 'building healthy alliances'). Thus it provides official support to the notion of community involvement in health.

The initial impetus for HFA 2000 came from demands for new approaches to health development in the Third World as increasingly, and certainly by the 1960s, a colonial model of health development was being questioned. However, it was soon linked to a perceived health crisis in industrialised countries: 'In the industrialised countries inequalities in health are increasing between social groups while health costs continue to rise. Moreover, the public interest in health, self-care and mutual aid has led to the questioning of professional approaches and definitions in health problems.'[3]

This stimulated the actions of those who sought to gain a recognition that a truly complete health promotion approach would require social and community action as well as individual behaviour change (Webster 1989, p. 3).

The HFA strategy stresses the importance of community participation in a number of documents:

It is a basic tenet of the Health for All philosophy that ... health developments in communities are made not only for but with and by the people. [WHO, *Targets for Health For All*,1985]

[Health promotion] is the process of enabling people to increase control over and to improve their health. ... At the heart of this process is the empowerment of communities, their ownership and control of their own endeavours and destinies. [*Ottawa Charter*, 1986]

Healthy public policy requires the means for informed public participation in priority setting, in strategic planning and in decision making. To succeed, such policy must be made by the public, for the public and in public. ['Creating Healthy Public Policy', WHO Conference in Adelaide, 1988]

Increasing community involvement in policy development should not lead to a situation in which the most educated, articulate and influential groups in society dominate the debate. Priority must be given to making the involvement of indigenous, disadvantaged and minority groups possible. [WHO 1988]

The 4th International Conference on Health Promotion held in Jakarta recently (1997) restated the importance of these elements of a Health For All strategy. The Jakarta Declaration on Health Promotion into the 21st Century stated that the need to 'increase community capacity and empower the individual' is one of the five priorities for health promotion (Scott-Samuel 1997).

Within the UK the HFA movement has been influential in a number of different ways. It has had an effect on the practice of many people active in the community health field at different levels, as representing both principles and practice which support community involvement in health. It has been heavily influential at structural level. In 1987, the WHO's European Office formally designated a number of European cities as 'Healthy Cities', of which four are in the UK: Camden (in London), Belfast, Liverpool and Glasgow. In addition many health authorities and local authorities have separately or together established local HFA strategies, often with a designated unit or member of staff to co-ordinate their development and the action associated with that. In turn this led to the establishment of the UK Health For All Network (UKHFAN) in 1987 as a membership organisation to act as a support for all those interested in taking forward the principles and practice of Health For All. The current role of this organisation is described in more detail in Chapter 2 under 'The growth of the community health movement'.

A number of local HFA units and projects have explicitly sought to promote and support community development around health, seeing this as an appropriate method as well as an important principle in achieving community participation in health. Some, such as Sheffield Health 2000 and Knowsley Health 2000, have developed clear community development and health strategies (Healthy Sheffield Support Team 1993, Labyrinth 1994a). Others have funded local community development projects, or provided local training in community development approaches to health, or set up community health forums and networks, or assisted in a variety of other ways (see various UKHFAN Newsletters).

Self-help

'Helping yourself' has long been a feature of community activity, with individuals seeking to improve their lot. As an activity, it becomes crucial to community involvement in health when it is organised on a group basis, that is, when individuals with the same or similar experience or problem come together for mutual support and help in tackling that problem. Self-help groups have been a feature of community life throughout this century and are an important part of organised community activity. Crucially, they are independent groups: they are run by their own members and are set up to serve their own interests. There are many examples, ranging from savings clubs to mother and toddler groups, to groups of those who share a common illness and so on. In terms of membership, they represent the largest section of the voluntary sector, and yet they are the least funded (Chanan 1991). Many receive no funds at all and do not require any, while others receive financial help in meeting the costs of a meeting place, childcare to enable involvement, publicity, transport to get to meetings and so forth. Some get some paid development support from an allied voluntary organisation (such as the Alzheimer's Society or MIND), while most have no contact with paid workers at all. None the less they have contributed to the shape of community involvement in health in many ways.

Self-help groups are a source of a particular consumer, user or community voice. They are health enhancing in their own right, as they provide support for and build the confidence and skills of their members. When they come together with similar self-help groups they represent an enormous depth of experience of a particular issue or problem, and can generate creative and effective ways of dealing with some of these. Some members of self-help groups gain confidence through membership, which enables and supports them in getting involved in wider community activity. These contributions have become particularly noticeable with the formation of 'user groups' which are a particular type of self-help group.

User groups are, as the name suggests, groups of people who define themselves as users of a particular service. Within the health field, such groups have come to prominence through the recent changes in Community Care, sparked off by the NHS and Community Care Act (1990). However, user groups already existed, particularly in the fields of mental health and learning disability, where people came together to share common concerns, often with the support of sympathetic professionals or campaigning voluntary organisations. As social services departments and health authorities now have a clear obligation to consult with users and carers, as well as with other bodies, on all aspects of community care, so many have seen the existence of user groups as a support in this process.

Many self-help groups have an explicit concern with health. In 1985 the Community Health Initiatives Resource Unit discovered that in the UK there were over 10,000 community health initiatives. Of these, self-help groups were by far the most numerous (Watt, 1986). In recognition of this fact a national Self-Help Resource Centre was set up by the National Council of Voluntary Organisations in the late 1980s, which then became independent. It acted as a source of advice and information to self-help groups and networks and maintained effective links with the community health movement.

Lobbying and campaigning

In this context, we define lobbying as attempts to influence the formulation of policy or legislation on behalf of a particular interest, and campaigning as a co-ordinated series of activities designed to meet a particular social or political goal. They can incorporate mass movements and demonstrations, such as the National Abortion Campaign, the Disability Rights Campaign or the Women's Peace Movement. Alternatively they can be very localised, as in the KAPIT community campaign in Kirkby on Merseyside (Kirkby Against Poisons, Incinerators and Toxins) (Labyrinth 1994a). Sometimes campaigns are set up to achieve a specific end and are disbanded once that end is achieved or abandoned. Commonly, however, they are one aspect of wider community activity. For example, many local Women's Aid groups are set up to provide a service for women; experience of providing that service has highlighted a number of gaps and discrepancies which has led the National Federation of Women's Aid to campaign explicitly to change policy, practice and legislation in the field of violence against women.

Traditionally, campaigning has probably been the hardest form of community activity and community development for statutory bodies to take on: often, of course, the campaigns have been geared specifically to achieving change within those organisations, which has not always gone down well with them. However, this activity has also helped to shape the nature of community involvement in health and so has its place within that movement. For instance, the KAPIT campaign mentioned above can now be seen as an important part of the local authority's Agenda 21 strategy and wider action to improve the local environment.

Conclusion

The early roots of community involvement in health embody both 'top down' and 'bottom up' activities. The former are represented by early charitable, philanthropic and government initiatives to promote self-help, as well as the later policy initiatives of the 1960s designed to tackle or divert social unrest through community development. The latter are represented by different social movements which have emerged throughout the century, articulating their members' concerns and taking action to meet them – often through setting up self-help groups, or lobbying and campaigning activities. At the same time sympathetic professionals and policy makers at local, national and international levels, as represented for instance in the new public health movement, and the international 'Health For All' movement, have been equally influential.

As a result, the direction that community involvement in health has taken historically within the UK has not been a linear one. Sometimes government initiatives have acted to 'control' or shape community health activities – it has, for example, been argued that the Home Office closed down the Community Development Projects in the early 1970s because it did not like the conclusions the projects came to regarding the ways forward for community development (Green and Chapman 1991). At other times a local government emphasis on community development as a major force for 'empowerment' has greatly facilitated 'bottom up' developments, for instance through offering support to the establishment of autonomous user forums. At the same time, community development approaches to health have been more successful and able to work at a greater pace, where relevant social movements with their associated networking structures have existed to support 'bottom up' activities.

Notes

1   Marjorie Mayo (1994) discusses the 'shifting concept of community': 'It is not just that the term community has been used ambiguously; it has been contested, fought over, and appropriated for different uses and interests' (p. 48).
2   A copy of the current Public Health Alliance charter is available from the organisation (see Appendix for address).
3   From *Health Promotion* (1987), 1(4), quoted by Wendy Farrant (1991), 'Addressing the Contradictions: "Health For All" and the Community Health Movement' in *'Roots and Branches': Papers from the OU/HEA 1990 Winter School on Community Development and Health*, Milton Keynes: Open University, p. 151.

2 Emergence and development of the community health movement

Summary

This chapter traces the development of an organised United Kingdom community health movement. It begins by exploring the early days of community health initiatives when the voluntary sector took a lead in both local level initiatives and in the establishment of a formal national structure for supporting community health initiatives. It moves on to explore how key players from local authorities and health authorities became involved, and describes the various stages in consolidating both national networking and a sense of a 'community health movement'. The chapter then describes the growth of statutory sector interest and involvement, and the diversification and eventual decline of a formalised, networked community health movement in the early 1990s. Finally, the chapter ends by looking at the ways community development and health work has continued to thrive at local levels throughout the 1990s and the re-emergence of a national profile and sense of community health movement in the latter half of the decade.

Early history

Some writers have traced the early roots of community development and health work back to initiatives such as the Peckham Project, an initiative set up in the 1930s in Peckham, South London, by doctors who felt that simply providing health care for the poor was limited (Pearse and Crocker 1985). They began offering sessions on nutrition, exercise classes, trips for children and so forth, from a special centre in the area. This early example of the establishment of a wider, health promotion/prevention approach to community health followed a similar philosophy to those described in relation to the development of settlements in the previous chapter. That is to say, the Peckham Project's roots were in philanthropic philosophy rather than empowerment models. Nevertheless, this work was very pioneering for its time and made connections between people's living conditions and lack of opportunities for a good diet, exercise and a good standard of living, and their ability to lead a healthy lifestyle.

The development of a national profile for Community Development and Health work

In the 1970s a number of community health initiatives began to emerge out of existing community development projects, but in particular out of the women's movement and black movements. These were almost without exception based within the voluntary sector. In 1986 the Greater London Council organised a conference, with support from the King's Fund, to explore innovatory work being undertaken, within health care, across London and beyond (London Strategic Policy Unit 1986). The conference featured writers, such as Lesley Doyle and Jeanette Mitchell, who were highlighting problems with our traditional ways of looking at health, and advocating new approaches to health at that time; health professionals who were voicing concerns about the limits of an approach to health which was wholly oriented around illness and health care, such as Patrick Petroni and Alex Scott-Samuel; pioneers campaigning for appropriate services for illnesses including sickle-cell disease and community-based women's mental health initiatives, such as Elizabeth Anionwu and Sue Holland, and advocates of new ways of working for health care professionals, such as Vari Drennan's work with health visitors and Debbie Clark and Adi Cooper's work to develop collective multi-disciplinary working in general practice. Amongst this diverse group of people were some of the workers and supporters of the newly emerging community health projects including Riverside in Newcastle upon Tyne, Wells Park in Sydenham, London, and the Tower Hamlets Health Project, London (all of which still survive today).

In 1981 the London Community Health Resource (LCHR) was established by the London Voluntary Service Council (LVSC) as a means of networking together community health initiatives across London. This was initially funded by the Greater London Council and the King's Fund and employed two part-time workers concerned with information and development functions. It was managed through a steering group which mostly comprised local level community health workers, but also some 'radical' NHS staff from disciplines such as health promotion and health visiting. The notion of health professionals who supported community development work as being 'radical' has not entirely disappeared even today, but the concept was still in common currency towards the end of the 1980s when a paper was produced arguing for the NHS to play an enhanced role in supporting community health projects in the UK (Blennerhassett et al. 1989). A diagram in the paper which maps contributors to the UK community health movement (which was at its peak at that time) still used the concept of 'radical health professionals' – that is, community development and health work was still a fringe issue within the NHS. A version of the diagram in that paper is reproduced here to highlight the early roots of CDH work.

The following year, the National Council for Voluntary Organisation's (NCVO) Inner Cities Unit researched and published a report called *Community Based Health Initiatives* (Smith 1982). It identified around 20 or so

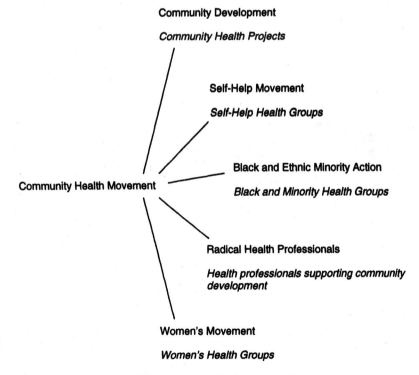

Figure 2.1   Some contributors to the UK community health movement (based on Blennerhassett et al. 1989, p. 200)

community health initiatives outside London, and recommended that NCVO follow up this research by seeking funding to establish a unit within NCVO to follow up this work, and to help support the development of new community health initiatives. In 1983 the Community Health Initiatives Resource Unit (CHIRU) was established, with funding through a Department of Health 'Section 64' Grant (voluntary sector funding). Three staff were appointed: an administrator, an information worker and a development worker. Their initial research identified many more initiatives than the 20 or so featured in the 1982 report. A national database was soon established, which included more than a thousand initiatives that identified with the term 'Community Health Initiative'. At this stage most of the initiatives were based in the voluntary sector.

Both LCHR and CHIRU continued their information and development work, and published a regular newsletter, *Community Health Action*. In 1986 the first national Community Development and Health (CDH) conference was held in Bradford (CHIRU/LCHR 1987a), attended by both voluntary and statutory sector workers and community activists (around two hundred people in all). It was clear that a thriving 'community health movement' was developing.

It became more and more obvious that the divide between London and the rest of the country was an arbitrary one, and increasingly LCHR and CHIRU worked jointly on projects and ventures. For example, the two organisations had overseen the development of a number of publications logging and debating developments in the community development and health movement (Kenner 1986, McNaught 1987). Both organisations were due for re-funding in the spring of 1987 and so it was decided to merge them and also to move away from the two national/London-wide host organisations. Later that year LCHR and CHIRU formally merged to become the National Community Health Resource (NCHR) and received re-funding through Department of Health 'Section 64' money for the new five-worker team. The two staff teams which had merged to form NCHR moved out of their host voluntary sector bases to form an independent voluntary organisation with its own membership, management committee and premises.

The development of a Community Development and Health 'social movement'

In 1987, *Guide to Community Health Projects* (CHIRU/LCHR 1987b) was published; it was intended as a resource document to help set out good practice guidelines for people in the process of setting up community health projects and as a guide to funders and those seeking funding. The publication was based on a survey of over 40 community health projects that were in existence at the time, drawing on the successes as well as the lessons that had been learned.

The next couple of years saw both a growth in membership of NCHR and increasing interest from the NHS and statutory sector workers in community development approaches to health. Specific issues were being raised by different sections of NCHR's membership. A national women's health conference was held in Harlow, Essex: over a hundred women from different parts of the country, many of whom were involved in women's health work in a voluntary capacity, came together at the two-day event. Although a number of organisations and networks already existed in relation to women's health, these tended to focus on particular health issues (such as cancer), or campaigns (for example, 'A Woman's Right to Choose' abortion campaign), or to be concerned with the exchange and distribution of health information, such as the Women's Health and Reproductive Rights Information Centre (WHRRIC). A wish to continue networking around issues in relation to the setting up and running of women's health groups and projects was expressed throughout the event. NCHR's development worker therefore set up the National Women's Health Network, which met quarterly in different parts of England.

Issues in relation to organising around black health issues were emerging from the wider community health movement too. There were a number of community health projects working specifically with black communities, and increasing numbers of black community health workers working within multi-racial environments. Further funding was secured from the King's Fund for a three-year post of Black Development Worker, and the national Black Health Forum was established, operating along similar lines to the National Women's Health Network.

The success in obtaining funding for a Black Development Worker encouraged NCHR to apply for funding for a full-time development worker to support the increasingly popular National Women's Health Network. By 1988 the Health Education Authority (HEA) had established a Women's Health Programme within the Professional and Community Development Division (PCD). A three-year grant was obtained from this programme to support a full-time development worker for the Women's Health Network, based at NCHR.

As well as responding to the needs and ideas for support from specific sectors of the community health movement, NCHR had also continued its wider role of general development and information work. A substantial library of resources including many unpublished reports from local projects as well as the growing number of NCHR in-house publications was gathered together throughout the 1980s. NCHR's base in London became a nationally recognised specialist information and resource centre which was regularly visited by researchers and academics from within the UK and further afield, as well as by many local workers and community activists anxious to learn from the community development and health work others were undertaking.

National conferences were another way in which the sense of a community health movement flourished. After the Bradford national conference in 1986 a second national conference was held in Salford two years later, attracting around 300 participants. Training was a major focus at this event, both in terms of the way it was organised, and in terms of the focus for workshop and plenary discussions. For the first time, facilitators were trained to support 'base groups' (random mixes of participants and specific self-selecting groups of participants, such as black women), who met three times throughout the event to look at training needs and ways of meeting them. Everyone who attended the conference had the opportunity to feed in their perspectives on training for community development and health work through the base group structure as well as attending a wide range of other workshops and discussions.

Following this event a regional structure was established to support community health workers across the UK to meet together for both informal networking and support, and more formal training sessions. However, it soon became clear that these evolving regional groupings would need some development time and financial resourcing if they were to grow and flourish. Funding was successfully sought from the Professional and Community Development Division of the Health Education Authority for two national training development workers to be based at NCHR. These posts supported the development of the Regional Training Networks across the UK, a national Training Working Party, and also linked in training issues and initiatives to the National Black Health Forum and National Women's Health Network. Thus by the end of the decade NCHR had developed from two small, time-limited, pilot projects (CHIRU and LCHR) into a well-established national voluntary organisation, with a large membership base, an active management committee drawn from around the country and a team of eight workers.

By the end of the 1980s the community health movement, and the initiatives and projects which were part of it, were still predominantly based outside mainstream NHS funding. Typically, initiatives received only short-term funding such as joint finance or inner-city partnership money and were usually run on a shoestring budget, often with just a single worker and a voluntary management group. In 1989 three people who were particularly involved with NCHR and in local level community health project work published an article which set out to make the case for the NHS supporting community health projects as part of mainstream activity. The sentiments expressed in the article are just as relevant today, despite nearly a decade of change in the NHS:

> There needs to be a systematic health authority policy for supporting CHPs, for example by grants, employment of workers with appropriate conditions of services, training of all health professionals in community development ways of working etc.
> This should go hand in hand with realistic policies for community participation, for example involving communities before decisions are taken, being open about planning so that the community has a chance to participate, setting up intersectoral planning forums. [Blennerhassett et al. 1989, p. 205]

The development of national health promotion involvement

A number of references have already been made to the Health Education Authority (HEA) in relation to national funding support for community development work. It is worth tracing the history of the Professional and Community Development Division (PCD) in order to understand subsequent developments in relation to the UK community health movement. The HEA was established as a special health authority in 1987 after the demise of the Health Education Council (HEC) quango. The woman appointed as the Director of the Professional Development Division was a well-known health promotion manager who had written and extensively advocated on behalf of community development approaches to health promotion (Adams 1991). Once appointed, she set about expanding the Division's remit to include community as well as professional development. An Assistant Director with responsibility for community development (CD) was recruited and a budget of £250,000 was moved across from professional development activities to support community development work. A women's health programme was established which was also managed by the Assistant Director: Community Development. The woman appointed to this post had been the National Development Worker for NCHR for the previous four years (and is also one of the authors of this book), so initially tight links were made between the newly established PCD Division and NCHR.

PCD Division set out to establish a national strategy for community development and health work from a statutory sector/health promotion agency perspective to complement and support the work undertaken by the voluntary sector at local and national levels. Although part of its aim was to increase statutory sector NHS understanding and support of community development and health work, it was important that the work was rooted in the needs of grass-roots community development and health workers and projects, and within the wider health promotion field. A series of regional workshops were held to look at how the HEA might best support local level work through its national level role and funding. The HEC had previously funded two local pilot community health projects in Mansfield (Mansfield CHP 1986) and Catford (Reason 1985), and work in relation to black health initiatives (HEC/THR 1985). However, although each initiative was successful in its own terms there was little impact on the national scene. It was felt important to avoid going down the route of funding pilot initiatives without a strategic plan and framework.

A definition of community development and health was drawn up and a strategic framework established. The strategic framework is set out below.

The main emphasis was on building a national infrastructure to support community development and health work (in partnership with NCHR). Such a partnership was seen as essential, as NCHR was an independent, membership-based organisation rooted in grass-roots community health work, whereas the HEA's accountability led back, via a Board appointed by the Secretary of State, to the Department of Health. As has been seen earlier in the chapter, some of the HEA's £250,000 yearly community development budget and some of the women's health programme budget was spent directly on bolstering up NCHR's role and activity by funding the training and women's health work. However, the HEA only had a remit for work across England, so meetings were established with the HEA's sister organisations in Wales, Scotland and Northern Ireland to seek their commitment and involvement in supporting community development and health work in their own countries as well as co-operatively across the UK.

Plans were made to establish a number of national initiatives (for example, training, policy), each with steering groups made up of PCD staff and local level workers and projects, to put the strategic framework into action in practical ways. However, within a few months of being established, the budget for CD work was frozen whilst the Department of Health reviewed whether CD was appropriate activity for the HEA (as an NHS statutory organisation) to be involved in. After three months the budget was freed up with the proviso that a formal evaluation be set in motion. However, the intervention by the Department of Health (D of H) gave the green card to those within the HEA itself who were sceptical about community development's effectiveness, or who felt it had a radical history and would therefore be a potentially disruptive influence within the organisation.

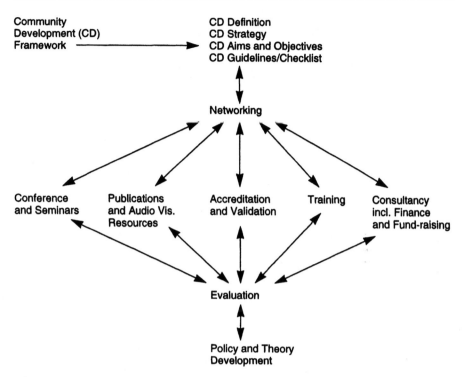

Figure 2.2   Health Education Authority community development infrastructure
(from *A National Strategy for Community Development and Health*, London: Professional and Community Development Division, Health Education Authority – unpublished document)

Community Development within the HEA survived for a further 18 months after the D of H review, but getting funding released for specific pieces of CDH work was always a struggle, even after the review freed up the overall CDH budget. Some senior-level opposition to notions such as 'women's health' and 'black health' remained entrenched and major differences over methodological and professional approaches to health promotion emerged within the organisation.

Evaluation methodology eventually proved to be the focal point for many of the internal disagreements. A struggle to reach an agreement to recruit a team of people with community development and health experience to undertake a review of the HEA's community development and health work was successful. The review took place under the co-ordination and academic management of the Open University; however their report was never published. It remained a document stamped 'Confidential – for limited internal circulation only' (Open University 1990). This is unfortunate as some of the methodology and findings were quite ground-breaking and would have been of interest to the community health movement and indeed wider health promotion and the NHS in general. A couple of the less controversial sections were eventually released by the HEA to the Open University for publication (Beattie 1991, Jones 1991). This particular aspect of HEA and community development and health history will be returned to later in this book when evaluation is explored in Chapter 10.

The growth of the community health movement

However, in 1989 the PCD Division was still alive and kicking, and the NCHR's national development and networking role continued to grow as did the funding of a number of initiatives that contributed towards the development of a national (that is, for England) strategy for CDH work, undertaken in partnership with (and funded by) the PCD division of the HEA. The third national conference was held in Newcastle in the autumn of that year and attracted 400 people; earlier that summer the second national Women's Health Conference was held in Liverpool and was attended by 200 women and 96 children. (The unexpectedly high cost of the crèche for this event also featured in the subsequent struggles over whether this sort of work was appropriate for the HEA.)

The UK Health For All Network (UKHFAN) (which started as networking between the four UK cities linked into the World Health Organization's European Office 'Healthy Cities' initiative and grew to be a national voluntary organisation with its own membership base and funding) was firmly established by the late 1980s. A 'Community Participation' sub-group of the main steering group was established in 1989. An average of twenty or so people from around the country began meeting together every three months to explore and develop work in relation to community participation in HFA and Healthy City type initiatives, and to ensure that the profile of this key principle of HFA was not lost in the large-scale multi-sector working that was emerging as an important approach to HFA in cities, towns and rural areas across the UK. The sub-group produced a paper putting forward ideas and guidance in relation to community participation in Healthy City/ Health For All type initiatives (UKHFAN 1991).

A number of publications in relation to CDH work were put together by the PCD, complementing earlier publications by NCHR. Unfortunately only one of these (Smithies and Adams 1990) had got as far as being formally published by the time CD and the HEA parted ways in June 1990; the other manuscripts never saw the light of day.

In the spring of 1990 the HEA organised the 'Roots and Branches Winter School', a week-long event which linked theory and practice, and academics with practitioners involved in community health initiatives. Experience of management and health professionals' lack of awareness of CD history and theory, both within the HEA and D of H at national levels, and local project experience at District Health Authority levels, showed that it was important to illustrate that community development and health work was rooted in sound theoretical and analytical models, and that work currently underway was critically written up and discussed. The event was the first of its kind in the UK. Funding was made available to encourage local-level project workers to write up aspects of their work critically and analytically rather than simply descriptively. Academics from fields that overlapped with community health work, but who had not had any real practical involvement, were encouraged to contribute papers which attempted to show how their academic discipline (for instance, social policy, social history, political science and so forth) could assist the development and analysis of community health work both in terms of theory and practice. The papers presented at the event were eventually released by the HEA for publication by the Open University (1991), though one paper which related to the HEA's CD work was withheld.

The decline of national support and co-ordination of Community Development and Health work

A month after the 'Winter School', just before publication of the Open University's review, mentioned above, the HEA decided (as part of an overall reorganisation) that the CD budget should be integrated into the organisation as a whole, rather than being a specific budget, and therefore a specific post to head up CD was also not needed. The Open University's review was very positive about the work that had been undertaken to date, but this did not change the management's position. Existing projects that were funded through the HEA carried on to the end of their pre-agreed funding period, but no further funding was made available after the late spring of 1990. Thus, as a result of the HEA's shift in priorities and policy, NCHR lost funding for the training and women's health parts of their work when their initial three-year contracts with the HEA ran out in 1991/92. The same period also saw the end of the King's Fund grant for development work with black and minority ethnic communities.

A national conference, held in Sheffield in 1991, was organised by a group of people involved with community development and health work across the country. The conference was funded through a small amount of money left over from a Yorkshire-based regional community development and health initiative, after it had ended prematurely. The event was entitled 'Community Development and Health: Reclaiming the National Agenda', and around 100 people attended (PHA 1992). The HEA (now minus the CD post and budget) and the remaining staff from NCHR were present, along with a representative from the UK Health For All Network's flourishing Community Participation sub-group. However, the majority of participants were from a range of local community health projects and initiatives. The aims of the event were:

- To re-establish the important contribution of CD to health at a national level.
- To debate issues of the last few years, looking particularly at the interconnections between the process of CD, local CD work and national support.
- To debate how the lobbying and campaigning aspects of CD and health could be taken forward, focusing on what support and resources were needed.
- To agree further action. [Webster 1992]

However, despite calls from the conference participants for the HEA to reinstate CD and for NCHR to align itself more closely with the needs and views of grass-roots community health workers and projects, there was no noticeable change in the priorities or actions of either organisation after the conference and thus no change at national level in terms of support offered to local level projects and workers.

In 1992 NCHR attempted to relaunch itself as Community Health UK. However, tensions about the low-key stance that NCHR had taken in relation to the HEA's withdrawal of funding from CDH nationally, and reductions and changes in staffing, meant that the previously active membership base began to fall away. The Department of Health 'Section 64' core grant was not renewed, and although Community Health UK continued to function in a small-scale way, its national impact was greatly diminished.

Shortly afterwards, Community Health UK organized a national conference in Preston in 1992, but it attracted fewer than 40 participants. The national archive of resources was removed from London to the local home-base of the director at that time, and is still housed there, in Bath. Small amounts of funding for specific project work have kept the profile of Community Health UK just above the horizon, and the *Community Health Action* magazine still comes out several times a year. However, the organisation is little known in the UK and appears to have little real credibility within community development and health fields.

That same year the UK HFA Network's national funding ceased. Subsequently, the organisation had to rely on membership fees and support from John Moores University in Liverpool, its host body. Economies were needed if the Network was to survive, and one of these was to change the post of national development worker into a more office-based administrator. The development worker had previously serviced and co-ordinated the Community Participation sub-group. Although the group continued to meet for another year or so, moving its meetings around the country and self-servicing, attendance eventually became so low that the few remaining active members decided that the meetings should cease.

Thus from its peak in 1989 when the community health movement had a strong national identity, was effectively networked in terms of specific interests (women's initiatives, black initiatives, and training), had a large and nationally accessible collection of archive and current materials and the support of both the HEA PCD Division and NCHR, there was a gradual (though at times accelerated) decline in support and networking which led to the demise of any sense of a common social movement.

By the late 1990s many of those involved in community development work at local level, and the wider NHS with its growing interest in community participation in health, know little if anything about the history that has been outlined in this chapter, and there is a huge sense of 'reinventing the wheel' as many of the debates and struggles of the 1980s, such as appropriate evaluation methods, the need for longer-term funding and the need for projects to be established with proper support and clear achievable objectives, are re-emerging.

Why did it all fall apart?

There are probably as many theories about why such a strong and relatively well-organised movement dissipated as there are people who were actively involved in the work at the time. Several points are worth reflecting on, however. First, for the first five or six years of its development, NCHR drew its staff predominantly from people who had previously been involved in community development and health work at local levels. As the organisation grew, people were recruited from wider health and voluntary sector fields, and some did not have a grounding in community development methods and approaches.

Second, during its period of growth in the late 1980s NCHR workers became more specialised and worked with particular sectors of the community health movement. This meant they had less of an overall view of the wider movement. In 1988 the generic national development worker post was replaced by a co-ordinator's post. The increased numbers of staff and complexity of the community health movement meant that significant amounts of the NCHR co-ordinator's time was taken up in internal management and the running of what was now quite a sizeable organisation with a reasonable annual financial budget to manage, rather than undertaking generic outreach and development work.

Third, when the HEA decision to absorb the CD budget and do away with a specialist CD assistant director level post (as part of their reorganisation) became known, NCHR did not take a public stance on the issue. Many community health workers organised separately to lobby the HEA and to try and gain media support for their arguments for keeping the budget and the post.[1] NCHR gradually, and for a number of different reasons, became distanced from the main groups and workers it was originally set up to support. Thus when its own re-funding came up for renewal many of its natural supporters had drifted away, and were not organised or concerned enough to fight for NCHR's survival. Community Health UK still exists, but its national profile within CDH is negligible, apart from the continued publication of the *Community Health Action* journal, which is now into its thirteenth year.

The reasons for the demise of community development and health work within the HEA are perhaps even more complex to unravel. Again, there are many different perspectives, including some who feel that the HEA did not abandon CD but merely re-oriented itself (Spray 1992). It is probably simplest to say that the ideas and ways of working that were being pioneered through the PCD Division were ahead of their time in terms of NHS and health promotion policy and practice. The Division achieved quite a lot in a relatively short space of time, but failed to convince many people within the HEA and the D of H that community development was a valid and appropriate activity to be engaged in. Its main support came from outside, rather than from within the HEA itself. The pace of change was such that it aroused suspicion and defensiveness at some senior management levels. Thus the 1990 HEA internal reorganisation presented an opportunity to reduce the profile of CD by integrating it into everyone's work (which effectively diluted it almost completely) rather than seeing it as a specialist area with its own specific budget.

Community Development and Health rises again

However, the overall picture for Community Development and Health is becoming more positive, and during the mid-1990s, the national profile of community health initiatives throughout the UK has been through something of a revival. Initiatives such as 'Local Voices' (NHSME 1992b) and 'Health of the Nation' (Dept. of Health 1992) in England and similar initiatives by the Scottish Office (1992) and the Northern Ireland Office (DHSS(NI) 1996), which stress the need to involve local people in health, have given a lift to CDH work at local levels, particularly through health purchasing agendas (Labyrinth 1996b).

The mid-1990s saw the re-emergence of national co-ordination in relation to CDH work – but not in England! Northern Ireland formally established, and gained European funding for, its own Community Development and Health Network in 1994 (and appointed a worker to co-ordinate this in early 1995). Health Promotion Wales initiated the 'Communities for Better Health Network' (which is still up and running, though not all of the initiatives that are members could be classed as 'community development' work). Scotland, through the Health Education Board for Scotland (HEBS), established a national post for community health in 1994 and held a national conference the following year, the first in Scotland to focus on CDH (Labyrinth 1995g). HEBS also surveyed the need for networking and co-ordination across Scotland (Labyrinth 1995h), and has recently funded a national development worker based within the voluntary sector to co-ordinate the Community Development and Health Network (Scotland) and to set up and administer a Scotland-wide database of community health initiatives.

Labyrinth Training and Consultancy (an independent organisation run by the authors of this book) organised and ran a national community development conference in 1995 entitled 'Moving On'. The event was held in Bradford (home of the first-ever national conference some ten years previously). The event attracted its capacity audience of 150, made up of people from both the statutory and voluntary sectors, and from geographical communities and communities of interest from around the UK. The conference report explores the focus and content of the event in more depth (Labyrinth 1995c). At the end of the event there was a demand for continuation of networking and support.

Currently, a number of initiatives emerging from the 1995 conference are continuing to support the development and resourcing of community health initiatives in the UK. The Standing Conference for Community Development (SCCD – a national voluntary organisation based in Sheffield) is supporting a number of regional networks for community development and health workers, and worked with Community Links (also a national organisation based in South Yorkshire) to produce an 'ideas' publication with practical examples of community health work (Community Links 1997). A network of people calling themselves the 'National Community Development and Health Network (England)' have been meeting since the conference, supported by SCCD and Community Links. A constitution and steering group have been established and various funding applications are being pursued to finance a national development worker, an information/administrative worker and an office, database and other support systems. A national conference took place in the autumn of 1997 (in Oldham) to launch the Network and the Community Links' publication.[2] The event was massively over-subscribed, which confirms the demand for national networking and support in England.

Funding is also being sought to set up and support a London community development and health network. When one considers the emergence of the London Community Health resource back in 1981, then one begins to get a clear picture of the somewhat circular nature of the community health movement.

The next chapter explores the ways in which current social and policy issues have implications for the recent rise of the Community Development and Health movement.

Box 2.1   Community Development and Health: 25 years of change

1970s & 80s: Local projects emerging out of Women's and Black movements

1981:   Development of London Community Health Resource (LCHR) (funded by King's Fund/GLC)

1982:   National Council for Voluntary Organisations (NCVO) Inner Cities Unit publish 'Community Based Health Initiatives'

1983:   Community Health Initiatives Resource Unit (CHIRU) established at NCVO (funded by Department of Health)

1986:   CHIRU and LCHR merge to form National Community Health Resource (NCHR)
First national Community Development and Health (CDH) Conference, Bradford

1987–8:	NCHR formally established as an independent voluntary organisation National Black Health Forum established National Women's Health Network established CDH Training Project established and Regional Training Groups set up across England Second National CDH Conference (Salford)
1988:	Health Education Authority (HEA) sets up Professional and Community Development (PCD) Division – £250,000 budget for CD, including some funding for NCHR
1988–9:	PCD Division attempts to establish a national (England) CDH strategy UK HFA Network's Community Participation Network launched
1989:	Third National CDH Conference (Newcastle)
1990:	'Roots and Branches' Winter School, organised jointly HEA and Open University HEA drops CDH as specific budget and post
1991–2:	'Community Development and Health – Reclaiming the National Agenda': National Seminar (Sheffield) NCHR loses HEA funding for Women's Health Network and Training Project NCHR loses funding for Black Health Forum Development Worker
1992–3:	Community Health UK (CHUK) established out of NCHR. CHUK loses Department of Health core funding
1994:	Northern Ireland establishes its own Community Health Network Scotland establishes community post at the Health Education Board for Scotland Health Promotion Wales establishes 'Communities for Better Health' Network
1995:	First Scottish Community Development and Health Conference

'Moving On' National CDH Conference in Bradford
CDH Network post for Northern Ireland

1996:   CDH post for Scotland
National CDH Network formed in England

1997:   Launch of CDH Network (England) & Community Links
CDH Ideas Annual

Notes

1   For example, see *The Lancet* (1990) 336, August 11, p. 363.
2   'Community Development and Health' Conference, September 1997, organised
by Community Links, Community Development and Health Network (England), and SCCD. Report 1998.

3 Bringing it up to date: social and policy issues

Summary

This chapter begins by looking at some of the government initiatives from the last ten years or so which have promoted the message that enabling community involvement in health is a legitimate and necessary activity for health and local authorities. It looks at the effects of the NHS and Community Care Act of 1990 in relation to community-based needs assessment, involving 'local voices' in commissioning, and the development of partnerships or 'healthy alliances'. It moves on to look at the policy initiatives which are just emerging from the Labour Government. Some of the social and policy issues, such as regeneration and the recognition of increasing health inequalities are then considered, which are affecting the way the public sector is promoting and responding to a growing public interest in health, along with the changing roles of local government and the voluntary sector in this regard. It also examines changes and developments within communities themselves, such as the development of the advocacy and user movement. Finally, the chapter discusses some new concepts that are encouraging the development of new ways of building and supporting infrastructures to sustain community involvement in health.

Central government initiatives

Chapter 1 described the role played by central government throughout this century in shaping and supporting the emerging community development movement within the UK. At different times both 'top down' and 'bottom up' approaches to this work have been highlighted and supported by government, while at other times government has seemed to ignore community development activity entirely. This apparently contradictory approach has continued to the present day. A number of government-led policy initiatives in the last ten years have had a direct impact on the growth and shape of community involvement in health. The most obvious one to start with, in so far as it relates directly and visibly to health, is the NHS and Community Care Act of 1990 and its associated documents and guidelines.

This Act has had a number of far-reaching consequences and we focus here on some of the consequences for community involvement in health. The changes in community-based care, co-ordinated by Social Services, has led to an increased emphasis on service user and carer involvement, and the development of advocacy initiatives. Many of the people involved in these groups and initiatives also have clear links and concerns about health issues as well as social welfare. Self-help and campaigning organisations and movements such as those coming out of the HIV/AIDS crisis (Prout and Deverell 1995) and the disabled people's networks (such as People First) have made sure that community health includes communities with common interests as well as those with shared geographical neighbourhoods. Chapter 7 on advocacy explores the links between CDH work and communities of interest in more depth.

One immediate effect of the Act was the separation of the health purchasing role of the new health authorities from the health care providing role of the new NHS Trusts, and the associated introduction and growth of GP fundholding practices. Whilst this was first introduced in England, it has since spread to the other countries of the UK. The Department of Health emphasised that the role of the new health authorities was to improve the health of their populations; that is, it was not limited to improving the quality or effectiveness of health care services. This emphasis was repeated again, to different degrees, in the four national strategies for health developed by government; 'Health of the Nation' (England), 'Scotland's Health: A Challenge to Us All', 'Health for All in Wales', and 'Health and Well-being into the Next Millennium' (Northern Ireland). These strategies allowed '[a]n opportunity to attend to broader public health issues which go beyond the responsibilities of the NHS' (Hunter 1993).

In 1997 a higher profile was seen for community development and participation work in relation to primary care. The King's Fund launched a publication on community development and involvement as part of its Community-Oriented Primary Care initiative (Freeman et al. 1997). The Public Health Alliance Trust (the charitable arm of the Public Health Alliance) commissioned work to explore a public health model of primary care. The model proposed by the researchers firmly links primary care with community development and participation (Peckham et al. 1997). A UK-wide conference, called 'Needs Assessment and Community Involvement in Primary Health Care' (organised by Labyrinth Training and Consultancy) was held in October 1997, and featured numerous examples of interesting practice from around England.

These developments were significant in relation to community involvement because they implied a formal recognition that the improvement of health was not solely the remit of the NHS and that other organisations and individuals have an important and crucial role to play in this regard. This recognition echoed an important aspect of the views and perspectives of both the 'New Public Health' and the 'Health For All' movements described in Chapter 1. It also implied that health authorities had a duty to engage and work with organisations and local people in their areas in order to influence and affect all the factors which have an impact on health. This was emphasised in the importance given to the role of health authorities as commissioners for health and as 'champions of the people'. In practice this led to a number of policy initiatives encouraging community development approaches to health within the NHS. They included the development of community-based health needs assessments, involving 'local voices' at every stage of commissioning and purchasing, and the development of 'healthy alliances' between organisations and groups. Their significance is described below.

Community-based health needs assessments

The move to commissioning status placed a clear obligation on health authorities to assess the health needs of their local populations. In the past this assessment was usually based on epidemiological surveys; and there continued to be an emphasis on gathering quantitative data which is used by Directors of Public Health in their annual reports to describe the health characteristics of their local populations in terms of morbidity, mortality, incidence of particular diseases and so on. In a new development, many health authorities have begun to seek the views of local people about their health and this has provided an opportunity to engage with local communities about issues that they see as affecting their health. Chapter 9 describes in detail a participatory approach to health needs assessment, with case studies and examples of useful models.

However, carrying out a community-based health survey has not inevitably led to community involvement in health. Sometimes such surveys have been seen as simple information-gathering exercises, with little thought or commitment on the part of the health authority to taking action to meet the needs identified by local people. In such cases the local people involved have become disillusioned and uninterested in engaging in any further discussion with the authority. Sometimes such surveys have thrown up issues which are outside the traditional remit of the health authority which may not, yet, have established effective links with those organisations which could act on these issues. In these situations it is difficult to sustain community involvement as local people do not see that they are gaining from the exercise. Equally, health authority representatives may not see the value of community-based health needs assessments if their organisation does not have the mechanisms, culture, organisational capacity or commitment to realise, take on and act on the implications of information gained through such surveys. In these situations it is not enough to carry out a participative survey. Some 'organisation development' within health authorities, and probably between health and local authorities, will be necessary to enable the existing culture and mechanisms to change and develop so that community views can be incorporated into decision-making structures affecting health. Chapters 11 and 14 describe the importance of organisation development to sustaining community involvement in health, and associated mechanisms, in more detail. However, community-based surveys can be seen as complementing and enriching the quantitative data gained through other sources. They can, for instance, explain why people act in a certain way and therefore what needs to change in order to enable them to act differently (NIHSS and PHRRC 1992). In many cases the requirement on health authorities to assess health needs has been an important vehicle through which community involvement in health has been enabled and supported and Chapter 9 explains how, and where, this can happen.

Local Voices

An essential element of community-based health needs assessments has been the Department of Health's 'Local Voices' initiative. In January 1992 the NHS Management Executive, as it then was, published a report which was to be extremely influential in the debate about community involvement in health. *Local Voices* (NHSME 1992b) set out its perspective in the preface:

> Making health services more responsive to the needs, views and preferences of local people is central to the new role of DHAs and FHSAs. The Patient's Charter, with its emphasis on people's rights under the NHS, reinforces the need for health authorities to seek people's views and to provide better information about health and health services.
>
> To give people an effective voice in the shaping of health services locally will call for a radically different approach from that employed in the past. In particu-

lar, there needs to be a move away from one-off consultation towards ongoing involvement of local people in purchasing activities. [p. 1]

The report then expands on the importance of local people's views:

There are a number of reasons for involving local people in the purchasing process. If health authorities are to establish a champion of the people role, their decisions should reflect, so far as practical, what people want, their preferences, concerns and values. Being responsive to local views will enhance the credibility of health authorities but, more importantly, is likely to result in services which are better suited to local needs and therefore more appropriate. There may of course be occasions when local views have to be over-ridden (e.g. on the weight of epidemiological, resource or other considerations) and in such circumstances, it is important that health authorities explain the reasons for their decision. [p. 3]

The report describes four essential activities which health authorities should engage in with regard to involving local people: listening, informing, discussing and reporting. It also describes a model of how arrangements to secure the views of local people fit into the purchasing process.

This influential report was followed shortly afterwards by a number of documents commissioned by the NHS Management Executive and designed to help health authorities make the changes suggested in the *local voices* report. They include the report on participatory survey and research methodology, *Listening to Local Voices* (NIHSS and PHRRC 1992) and the report on training and organisation development implications for health authorities, *Responding to Local Voices* (Labyrinth 1993b). This latter report, which was based on research with a number of different district and regional health authorities, found that while a number of authorities were grappling with the requirements of *Local Voices*, it tended, at this stage (1993) to be in an *ad hoc* way. What was clearly needed, argued the report, was a strategic commitment to community involvement; and it suggested a number of ways in which this could happen. These are described in detail in Chapters 12 and 14.

Shortly afterwards the then Minister for Health outlined what the seven main 'stepping stones' to successful health purchasing were. They gave a clear message that community involvement in health needed to be addressed at the strategic level, as 'responsiveness to local people' was seen as one of the seven steps, along with a clear strategy, effective contracts, building an informed knowledge base, building mature relations with providers, building organisational capacity for change and building local alliances for health (NHSME 1993). He followed this up in the following year with a number of statements designed to make clear to health authorities that involving local people needed to be a continuous, strategic and measurable purchasing activity at all levels:

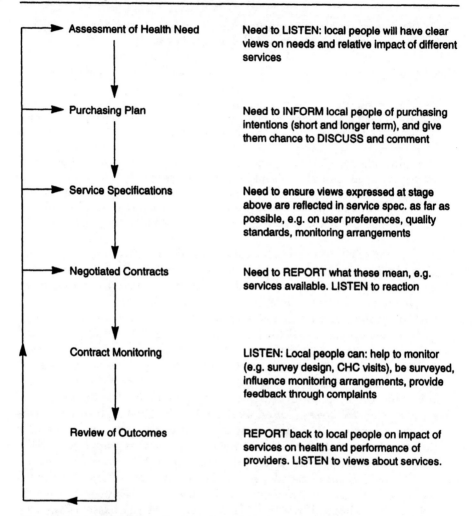

Figure 3.1   Making local voices heard in purchasing for health (NHSME 1992b, p. 16)

We must get away from the notion that health services can be designed for the community by 'experts' who define people's needs, but ignore their wishes. Health authorities must demonstrate that they are going the extra mile to explain their proposals, to take account of people's concerns and to carry the public with them. [Department of Health 1994]

The message from the Department of Health about the importance of 'local voices' and community involvement was clear, and a number of gains have been made in this connection. However, at local level, many health authorities still have a long way to go to make this involvement a reality. A national workshop, 'Local Voices: Three Years On', held in July 1995 and attended by those responsible for 'local voices' work within health authorities, came up with a number of issues that still need addressing. At organisational level, there is still a need for greater co-ordination of 'local voices' work strategically, with associated resources and training for staff in the new skills required. Equally it was felt important to maintain a 'bottom up' approach and steer clear of token exercises, while continuing to build the vision and commitment to change within health authorities. At community level, there is a continuing need to audit what is already going on so that health authorities do not 'reinvent the wheel', to feed developmental resources to communities and to develop and maintain a two-way dialogue with communities. Participants also stressed the need for a partnership/inter-agency approach to 'local voices' so that the process, outcomes and necessary action can be commonly owned and shared. Finally it was expressed strongly that central government needs to continue to give top-level support to 'local voices' work and clear messages to health authorities and boards that this work remains a priority (Labyrinth 1995b).

Healthy alliances

Building local alliances for health was one of the Department of Health's seven 'stepping stones' to successful purchasing, as described above, as well as one of the key principles of 'Health For All', for all the four national health strategies within the UK. For example, in one of the documents, Health of the Nation (1993), the Department of Health describes its rationale for promoting 'healthy alliances' in the following way:

Approaching the 21st century, the greatest advances in health will come in three main ways:

- encouraging people themselves to lead healthier and safer lives and promoting the availability of affordable healthy choices – changing behaviour;
- ensuring healthier and safer environments in which people can live, work and play – changing environments; and
- providing the right type of high quality local services – providing better services.

These can be achieved most effectively when individuals, groups and organisations work together through recognising the common ground between them and agreeing on shared objectives.

This document also clearly outlines the advantages of healthy alliances as being a more effective use of resources, broadening responsibility for health, breaking down barriers/building knowledge, exchange of information, developing local health strategies, generating networks and developing seamless services (Health of the Nation 1993, p. 22). There are a number of government-sponsored reports which provide practical suggestions on how to set up, maintain and evaluate healthy alliances (NHSME 1992a, Health of the Nation 1993, NHSTD 1993b, Funnell et al. 1995, Powell 1992). However, while alliance working between organisations is clearly an important part of action to improve health, it does not necessarily lead to greater community involvement. On the one hand, voluntary organisations were increasingly recognised as key players within healthy alliances (Health of the Nation 1993, pp. 41–42). On the other hand, many health authorities (as well as local authorities) do not see a distinction between 'voluntary organisations' and 'local people', and so act as though the involvement of voluntary organisations in a healthy alliance equates with the involvement of local people. Clearly there is a link; for instance, many Councils of Voluntary Service have contacts with, develop and support a number of community-based groups. Voluntary organisations, on the whole, work for local people, providing services for them, and do not claim to represent local people. However, they can provide a valuable and skilled path to the enormous number and broad range of local, self-help, user and community groups which exist in an area and thus play a key role in enabling community involvement within an alliance. It is, however, very important to note that community involvement in health can be enabled through a healthy alliance and begins, rather than ends, with the involvement of voluntary organisations in such an alliance.

Changes introduced by the Labour government

The Labour government, elected in May 1997, has wasted little time in bringing forward policies to reform and develop the NHS and work to promote the health of the UK population. The White Paper *The New NHS. Modern. Dependable* (Department of Health 1997) sets out many changes and developments from the 1990 Act introduced by the Conservative government. It remains to be seen how many of these will impact community involvement in practice, but the document certainly includes statements that can be seen as favourable. Separate documents on the future of the NHS have also been launched for each of the other three UK countries. The introduction to the English White Paper contains the following statement:

Openness and public involvement will be key features of all parts of the new NHS. [p. 15]

There will be a new NHS Charter, replacing the Patient's Charter. The NHS Executive will be given the role of supporting the range of initiatives in the White Paper on greater involvement for the public, patients and carers. This includes work in relation to developing the capacity of Regional Offices, NHS Trusts and Health Authorities to undertake public involvement and partnership working, as well as involving users and carers in the NHS Executive's own work programme (p. 62). Health authorities are to be given four specific roles in relation to communicating with local people and ensuring public involvement in decision making. These include participating in a new national survey of patient and users experience, and ensuring public involvement in their local Health Improvement Programme and Primary Care Groups (see below).

A new national performance framework will be developed focusing on six areas of performance. These are:

1 Health improvement.
2 Fair access.
3 Effective delivery of appropriate health care.
4 Efficiency.
5 Patient/carer experience.
6 Health outcomes of NHS care.

All the dimensions set out above can be usefully tied in to community involvement in health, but some are directly relevant. Dimension 2 (fair access) used as an example, ensures that black and minority groups are not disadvantaged in terms of access to services. Dimension 5 (patient/carer experience in relation to the quality of treatment and care) is also particularly useful in the context of community involvement in health work.

'Healthy alliance' work is given a formal boost by introducing statutory duties of partnership for health authorities, local authorities and NHS Trusts. The role of local authorities in health is given strong prominence in several sections of the document. Each health authority will be required to develop a local Health Improvement Programme to provide a framework within which all NHS organisations can operate. Such programmes 'will identify the health needs of local people and what needs to be done about them' (p. 24). Programmes will be developed in partnership with other NHS bodies, local authorities, academic and research interests, voluntary organisations and local communities. The first programme will start in April 1999 and set a three year plan which will be reviewed annually. The programme will be progressively updated.

The move to introduce Primary Care Groups led by GPs and community nurses, serving populations which are deemed to be 'natural communities' (p. 37), should bring decision making and access to resources closer to local communities. All Primary Care Groups are required to have clear arrangements for public involvement, including open meetings (p. 36). They will be 'encouraged to play an active part in community development and in improving health in its widest sense' (p. 39).

The Health Action Zones (HAZ) initiative, which has been established 'to explore new, flexible, local ways of delivering health and health care' (p. 76) will initially target twelve areas of the country in regions of 'pronounced deprivation' (p. 77). 'The accent will be on partnership and innovation, finding new ways to tackle health problems and reshape local services' (p. 77). The White Paper states that 'Health Action Zones will offer opportunities to explore new ways of involving local people' (p. 29). All successful HAZ bids will have to illustrate community involvement and public accountability.

The Government has also launched a Green Paper *Our Healthier Nation* (Department of Health 1998) which replaces *Health of the Nation* in England. Similar documents have been launched for Scotland, Wales and Northern Ireland. (The Northern Ireland document is particularly strong on community development.) The paper sets out a national strategy for improving the public's health, and seeks to highlight and find ways to address health inequalities. The summary document released by the Department of Health (1998) notes 'a key priority is improving health for those who are worse off' (p. 1). The effects of social, environmental and economic factors on health are highlighted, alongside the effects of an individual's lifestyle. Again a 'partnership' approach is put forward.

> While people on their own can find it hard to make a difference; when individuals, families, local agencies and communities and the Government work together deep seated problems can be tackled. [p. 3]

Voluntary organisations are said to have a role in acting as advocates to give a powerful voice to local people. Healthy neighbourhoods are highlighted as a key setting (with particular emphasis on older people) along with workplaces and schools. When the Green Paper progresses into formal policy it will undoubtedly provide a very useful and high profile context for community development based approaches to health promotion and public health.

Regeneration initiatives

Central government has been actively involved in regeneration since the late 1960s when it developed its Urban Programme. Both Conservative and Labour administrations have initiated action on regeneration; recent administrations have placed responsibility for overseeing regeneration within the Department of the Environment. Initial concerns were with physical and economic regeneration, and spending on housing, job creation and capital investment remain a major element of all regeneration programmes. There has, however, been a growing realisation at government level that regeneration will not be sustainable without the involvement of local communities at all levels of the programme. A number of research reports, most recently *Made to Last* (Fordham 1995), published by the Joseph Rowntree Foundation, make this point very clearly, based on evidence from a number of previous regeneration programmes. Therefore the most recent government programme, the Single Regeneration Budget (SRB), outlines more clearly than ever before that local authorities and other regeneration partners must seek, demonstrate and implement community involvement at every level, from making the bid to carrying out successful programmes. At the same time, community involvement is an essential element of application for regeneration funding from the European Commission.

The 1997 SRB Challenge Fund lists seven key objectives, of which one or more should be met through proposed bids. One of these objectives explicitly mentions health: 'to enhance the quality of life of local people, including their health and cultural and sports opportunities' (Department of Environment 1995, p. 2). The other six objectives are concerned with employment, economic growth, the environment, housing, community safety and benefiting ethnic minorities. SRB emphasises partnerships: local authorities are expected to have a central role, but *real* involvement of other private, public, voluntary and local community sectors is required. The supplementary guidance issued in July 1997 stressed that proposals should contribute to a commitment to carry out a concerted attack against the multiple causes of social and economic decline, including public health; have a greater emphasis on tackling the needs of communities in the most deprived areas, and illustrate a more collaborative approach.

The implications for community involvement in health are at least twofold. First, health is now considered a key element of regeneration. This unlocks resources, through the SRB Challenge Fund, which can be used to promote health initiatives in local areas. It also gives an added impetus to the creation of healthy alliances between organisations, and an accepted framework within which local and health authorities can work together and with other organisations and groups, to improve health. Second, it makes community participation a requirement of funding, rather than an optional extra. This is clearly spelt out in a number of publications from the Department of the Environment. For example:

> Local people can be involved in regeneration programmes in many ways either as individuals, through groups of various kinds including community groups, workplace groups or through their businesses. 'Professional' voluntary organisations play a role in local regeneration, often helping local people develop their skills or running projects. But they are not the same as local people and cannot substitute for them. ...
>
> For Challenge Fund ... there should be a significant degree of joint working between official agencies, community organisations and other partners. All partners should have an effective say in the allocation of resources and there should be effective arrangements to ensure that those sections of the community intended to benefit do so. [Department of the Environment 1995]

Both local people and health authorities have seen the benefits of getting involved in regeneration programmes. For instance, some health authorities have commissioned participatory health needs assessments and associated work to build community infrastructures and carry out internal organisation development, as part of SRB bids and programmes, for example, such as North Staffordshire Health Authority (Labyrinth 1995f). Some local community groups have become actively involved in initiating and developing local health strategies for their SRB area for example, Speke and Garston Health Development Project in Merseyside is part of an SRB programme. A recent conference of people active in community development, sponsored by the Department of National Heritage, expressed the view that health needed to be kept as a central concern within all partnership initiatives, including regeneration.[1]

Increasing health inequalities

The need to 'redress inequalities in health' is a key principle of the international 'Health For All' movement, and the concern of many within the UK at local and national levels. However, it is only in the last few years that central government has, once again, recognised the existence of such inequalities and begun to address them as legitimate concerns.

The issue of inequality in health got very little coverage within NHS circles until the publication of the Report of the Working Party on Inequalities in Health (the 'Black Report') in 1980. This report particularly highlighted the relationship between social class and ill health. However, official public health response to this report was minimal and it was not until more than a decade later that this issue began to be taken seriously within the mainstream NHS (Webster 1992). Margaret Whitehead (1992) describes the 'hundreds of new studies' which illustrate the 'health divide' in a number of different ways, showing that 'better health' is experienced by the more advantaged in society. She describes differences in morbidity between socioeconomic groups, differences in social and mental health, health differentials between groups of different origin and so on. She identifies three determinants of ill health: health hazards in the physical and socioeconomic environment, inadequate access to health care and behavioural risk factors and barriers to changing personal lifestyle. The distribution of these determinants is uneven within the UK, with a heavier burden falling on more socially disadvantaged groups. She suggests that this unequal distribution is avoidable if health policies are designed around three aims: a direct attack on the determinants of the health divide, indirect attack by ameliorating the damage to health caused by the determinants and matching services to increased need. Richard Wilkinson (1992) has extended this argument by uncovering evidence which suggests that income distribution – of relative income rather than absolute income – is a fundamental determinant of national standards of health. That is, the health of the total population of a country grows worse as the income distribution within that country becomes more unequal; and vice versa.

In 1995, two quite different documents were published which have had a major effect on both legitimising the recognition of growing inequalities in health within the UK, and on generating action to address those inequalities. The first was published by the Public Health Alliance and is an extensive 'toolbox' for all those living and working in the area of poverty and health (Laughlin and Black 1995). The pack provides comprehensive information on the nature and causes of poverty and its links with ill-health. Its main focus is on providing material, models, ideas and examples of good practice designed to take action to tackle poverty and health. The second document was published by the Department of Health and talks about 'variations in health' rather than 'poverty' or 'inequalities'; but it addresses itself explicitly to the question of 'what can the Department of Health and the NHS do?' (Health of the Nation 1995).

Each of these influential reports emphasises the importance of the role of community involvement in tackling inequalities (or 'variations') in health. The Department of Health report states:

> Given the many and complex factors which contribute to variations in health, the importance of alliances, at both national and local level, cannot be overstated.

Genuine progress will depend on the involvement of other government departments, local authorities, the voluntary sector, and individuals and communities themselves. The Department of Health and the NHS have a particular

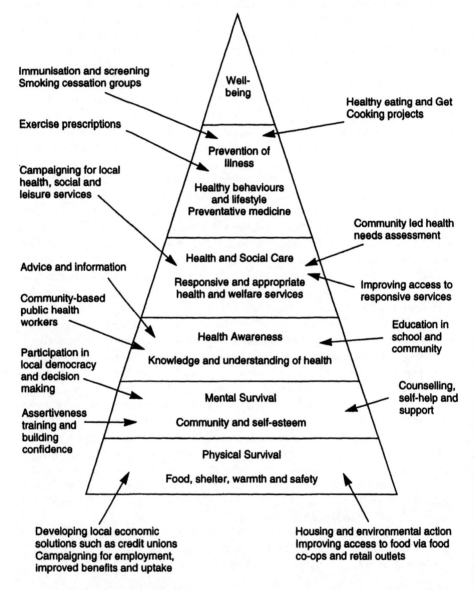

Figure 3.2   Hierarchy of health outcomes and examples of activities which develop them

responsibility in drawing attention to the need for such alliances and providing leadership and support. [Health of the Nation 1995, p. 2]

The Public Health Alliance pack is focused at community level and so most of the action it describes as tackling poverty and health is about community involvement to some degree or other. The diagram opposite is taken from the pack and gives examples of community involvement activities which address different layers of the factors which influence health. The pack states that:

> ... good health or well-being is reached via a number of hierarchical stages or outcomes. Activity focused at the top of the triangle will not lead to good health without activity also focusing at the bottom levels, and the balance of activity needs to reflect the characteristics of the local community.
>
> In poor communities, where the pre-requisites for physical survival are in doubt, promoting health needs to concentrate on work at that level. However even in areas where poverty is widespread, not everyone suffers to the same extent and the ideal way of responding to poverty and health issues in a community is to try and cover all the different levels of the hierarchy at the same time. [Laughlin and Black 1995, p. 42]

The change to a new Labour Party administration in Government has already led to clearer directives to link health improvements with reductions in inequalities; a new wider-ranging 'Health Strategy' has been proposed by Tessa Jowell MP, the new Minister for Public Health (which is itself a new post), and Frank Dobson MP, Secretary of State for Health has implemented the Government proposal to set up new 'Health Action Zones' which will link health and regeneration more closely.

An independent inquiry into health inequalities, chaired by Sir Donald Acheson, is due to report its findings in 1998. This may lead to the setting of specific targets in an attempt to reduce health inequalities.

The changing face of local government

The involvement of local authorities in health is not new. Until fairly recently the local Medical Officer for Health, as they were then called, was based within the local authority, and even now the local Director of Public Health, as they are now called, has clear links into the local authority although based within the health authority. Environmental health continues to lie within local authority control. 'Health For All' units are just as likely to be based within the local as within the health authority. As we have seen, local authorities are seen as key players by the Department of Health within any healthy alliance. In addition they provide the other key partner, along with the health authority, in joint funding and joint finance initiatives.

At the same time, the role of local government has changed within the last ten years. They are now required by central government to become 'enablers' rather than providers of local services. They, like health authorities and trusts, are part of the movement away from direct public provision of services towards an increasingly 'mixed economy of welfare', represented by the substantial use of market mechanisms as applied by service managers, as well as the increasing use of private and voluntary/not-for-profit agencies as service providers. This raises particular issues for community involvement. First, it requires local authorities to work in new ways, in partnership with the voluntary sector as well as the private sector. Increasingly, the voluntary sector is recognised as comprising a number of different elements, the largest of which is represented by informal community activity and community organisations, as well as the less numerous elements of more formal voluntary bodies. Thus, for such partnerships to be effective, local authorities have had to consider mechanisms which engage the more informal community-based and diverse groups, as well as the more formal ones. Second, the processes of local authorities contracting out their services depends on closer involvement of local communities, both in terms of developing service specifications and in terms of monitoring service delivery, whether the provider is from the statutory, private or voluntary sectors.

In a recent publication, *Local Authorities and Community Development* (Association of Metropolitan Authorities 1993), it is argued that many local authorities have found it easier to take on their new enabling role in a pro-active way where community development has been central to their work. This has enabled them to develop pro-active strategies such as these:

- Local authorities have developed new ways of working, as 'enabling authorities' in partnership with communities and community organisations.
- Local authorities have developed localisation and decentralisation strategies to bring them closer to the communities which they serve.
- Local authorities have developed strategies to democratise the planning and delivery of community services.
- Local authorities have developed strategies for quality services, working in partnership with their own staff and trade unions, and with users, user groups, carers and other community organisations.
- Local authorities have continued to develop equal opportunities policies, both in relation to their own staff and services and in relation to staff and services in the voluntary and community sectors. [Association of Metropolitan Authorities 1993]

So on the one hand, local authorities have a key role to play in influencing health. They are responsible, directly, or through contracting, or through strategic intervention, for a number of services which affect health including community care, housing, environmental services and so on. They are major players in initiating and developing key strategies which impinge on people's health, such as anti-poverty strategies, regeneration strategies and so on. On the other hand, as an 'enabler' the local authority 'is a natural broker and co-ordinator and a focus for partnership at local level; it can mobilise public opinion and take a holistic view of the local environment' (Hunter 1993). It has a vital role to play in developing community involvement.

Within this context the international 'Health For All' movement has several suggestions to make concerning the role of local government in facilitating community involvement in health, based on work with a 'healthy cities' focus. The World Health Organization (1988) defines a healthy city 'as one that is continually creating and improving those physical and social environments and expanding those community resources which enable people to mutually support each other in performing all the functions of life and in developing their maximum potential'. It also argues that this requires a 'healthy local democracy'. This notion of 'continually providing' places an emphasis on process and on ongoing involvement of the people in matters of local government.

This concern for an ongoing process of involvement in local government is given shape in the notion of 'governance'. Governance is defined as: 'the process by which we collectively solve our problems and meet our society's needs'. As such, it is distinct from 'government', which is the instrument we use. The instrument is outdated and the process of reinvention has begun.[2] Within this scenario it is suggested that the structure of local government has to be reorganised (or 're-invented') to deal with issues such as safety, sustainability, equity and so on, which cut across traditional local authority departments; this structure must be managed with a style that emphasises collaboration, negotiation and holistic approaches, rather than competition, hierarchy and sectoral approaches. At the same time it is seen as vital that the community is sitting round the table with the planners and policy makers, rather than kept to the margins.[3] It seems that there are some connections between what is happening within local government in the UK and some of the findings of the 'healthy cities' movement; both, at least, see a key role for local government as 'enablers' and facilitators of community involvement in health.

The new role of the voluntary sector

The voluntary sector within the UK is vast and encompasses an enormous range of different types of groups and organisations. Its history is as long as that of community development and comprises a similar mix of philanthropic and self-help tendencies (see Chapter 1). The extent and scale of voluntary sector activity varies enormously. A report by the National Council of Voluntary Organisations (NCVO 1990) distinguishes a number of broad areas of activity to describe the work of voluntary organisations. These are: service provision, self-help or mutual aid, advocacy and campaigning, and intermediary bodies (such as local development agencies, or umbrella organisations) who exist to help provide services to existing voluntary organisations and to develop new ones. The vast majority of government funding for the voluntary sector, locally and nationally, is directed at the first category of activity – service provision. Another report from the Health Education Authority (1992) identified a variety of ways in which voluntary sector organisations were involved in health promotion work. These included: training, campaigning and advocacy, access, self-help, information and education, policy development and service provision.

Research carried out by the Community Development Foundation (Chanan 1991) suggests that independent local community groups are the largest and least funded part of the voluntary sector. These groups arise primarily from community activity, not from the activities of national voluntary organisations. The report argues that at local level, the voluntary sector is an interdependent mixture of voluntary organisations and informal community groups. Furthermore, the ability and capacity of the established voluntary sector to reach and involve local people rests partly on informal community activity. Thus increasingly the voluntary sector is more accurately renamed 'the voluntary and community sector'.

The voluntary sector, like the NHS and local authorities, has been greatly affected by central government policy changes and initiatives, which in turn has had implications for their role in taking forward community involvement in health. Traditionally, the voluntary sector has enabled this involvement in a number of ways. The first community development and health projects in the UK in the 1970s were funded by charitable bodies, not the state, and placed within the voluntary sector (see Chapter 2). Any national or regional structures set up to support and promote community involvement in health, such as the Community Health Initiatives Resource Unit, the National Community Health Resource, the Community Health Network of the Standing Conference on Community Development, or the Northern Ireland Community Development and Health Network, have been based within the voluntary sector, although often funded from central or local government funds and sometimes supported by statutory sector workers. Today, community development and health workers are as likely to be employed by voluntary organisations as by the NHS or local authorities. Therefore the new roles of the voluntary sector have an impact.

Privatisation, the creation of non-departmental government bodies and the contracting out of public services have all created new partners for voluntary organisations to work with (NCVO 1990, p. 19). Voluntary organisations are also being encouraged to seek out new resources for their work, for example, bids for the National Lottery, SRB, European Community funds. In particular, the 'contract culture' has brought new issues to be faced. Research by Birmingham Settlement, an independent charity in inner-city Birmingham, suggests that there is an urgent need to maintain solidarity with other voluntary organisations and groups while competing for contracts (Kunz et al. 1989). Yet they see advantages in the new contracts: contracting can help increase the amount of control by the community over public services; it can enhance the ability of voluntary organisations to represent the interests of their constituency effectively, and it can lead to a more needs-related provision of public services.

At the same time it is argued that the contract culture treats the voluntary sector purely as a means of service provision. It ignores the continuum with independent community activity and threatens to drive a wedge between the two. Gabriel Chanan (1991) argues that: 'Contract culture is only half a policy for the voluntary sector. It needs to be paralleled by a separate funding and development stream to assist independent community activity' (p. 1). It seems that this message is beginning to get through to central government. Responsibility for community development at central government level was shifted recently (1996) from the Home Office to the Department of National Heritage, accompanied by a shift in name from the 'Voluntary Services Unit' to the 'Voluntary and Community Division'. Although it has now been shifted back to the Home Office the Division has kept its new name. The Division is currently carrying out research for the government, aimed at answering three very relevant questions: what are the preconditions for successful partnership between local communities and external agencies? What is the best form of investment that funders can make in communities? What lessons can be drawn from current community projects and how can these lessons be spread and applied? The ways in which these questions are addressed and responded to by local and national government will have a considerable impact on the support available for independent, informal community activity and involvement around health.

Advocacy and user involvement

We have seen in Chapter 1 how the advocacy and user involvement movement which has evolved in the last ten years in the UK has enabled many
groups who have traditionally been excluded from community activity, and
certainly from participation in the affairs of public bodies, to get involved
and stay involved. The impetus for this has been twofold. On the one hand
'users' themselves have become more assertive and organised about expressing their views. This has been particularly so in the field of mental
health and of learning disabilities, but has spread to all other 'categories' of
user. They have set up their own user or advocacy groups, sometimes with
the support of sympathetic voluntary organisations such as MIND or People First. On the other hand, the NHS and Community Care Act (1990)
referred to earlier has led to some statutory sector support for the movement. The Act places a duty on social services departments and health
authorities to consult with users and carers (as well as voluntary organisations) at every level of drawing up, implementing and reviewing policies,
strategies and practices in community care.

Recent research into user and carer involvement in community care shows
that the last few years has seen significant changes in policy, planning,
attitudes and services as a result of that involvement (Labyrinth 1995e).
What emerges from the large number of reports and publications which
seek to map activity and thinking as well as determine good practice is that
there is a need to approach user and carer involvement strategically. Chapter 14 explores this in more detail. There is also a degree of consensus that
user and carer involvement needs to be seen, and taken forward, within a
wider framework of public and community involvement.

The same research gives examples of many of the practical ways in which
health or local authorities are supporting advocacy and user involvement.
Some have set up User Forums, resourced by development workers; some
have set up specific carer or user groups, such as young carers' groups, as
self-help groups but with outside support. Others have supported advocacy groups within a particular service, or a scheme for independent advocates for individuals. Some have funded or contracted user and/or carer
groups and organisations to run and develop their own service.

Many of these initiatives relate equally to the NHS and to local authorities. Although many of them come under a 'community care' banner, they
inevitably feed into and inform the development of initiatives to promote
community involvement in health. A key feature of the effect they have had
has been the emphasis now placed on 'independence' within advocacy.
These movements around advocacy and user involvement have helped to

articulate in a very clear way that support for community involvement has to be independent, and independence is a key principle of the advocacy movement. Practically speaking, this is the notion that 'users' will only get involved in a way that empowers them, if at the very least their views and perspectives are listened to in their own right, without being subsumed under an agency agenda.

Developing sustainable infrastructures

The word 'sustainability' is heard increasingly in discussions of community involvement in health. It is used in at least two separate, though interlinked, ways. First, there is the economic sense of 'sustainable development'. In 1987 the World Commission on Environment and Development defined sustainable development as 'Development that meets the needs of current generations without compromising the ability of future generations to meet their needs' (p. 8). The link between this concept and health lies in the implication that any model of economic development and economic activity which 'looks to the future' will also be helpful in securing the health and well-being of the current generation (Crombie 1995, p. 1). A recent report from the Public Health Alliance, arising from a project on sustainable development and health, describes a number of principles which should underlie all health, environmental and economic activities and which are relevant to community involvement:

- Patterns of living and consumption must occur within sustainable limits.
- Economic activity is not an aim in itself but a method of benefiting people.
- It is important to empower communities in order to safeguard their health.
- Health, and consequently environmental qualities, should be a basic human right. This implies a corresponding duty to avoid damaging the environment of others, including both those at a distance and those not yet born. [Crombie 1995, p. 22]

Empowerment, rights and duties are all mentioned here and an effective method of putting these into practice is through community development. Community involvement is, in fact, a key element of the international action plan designed to bring about sustainable development for the twenty-first century, known as Agenda 21. This agenda was endorsed by over 150 nations at the Earth Summit in 1992 and includes plans for involving people at all levels in environmental action, in all nations. A workshop was run on this issue at 'Moving On', the national community development and health conference in 1995 (Labyrinth 1995c). Participants at this workshop concluded that both community workers, working at grass-roots levels, as well as health and local authority managers who work at more strategic levels, need to be encouraged to make links with Agenda 21 as having great implications for community involvement in health. As they say: 'Taken steadily, with many small practical steps shaped by local citizens, the programme has the potential to educate people and involve them in the bigger questions about our joint future' (Labyrinth 1995c, p. 4).

Secondly, sustainability is recognised as a key requirement of regeneration. The influential Joseph Rowntree Foundation report on creating sustainable regeneration, which considers the historical range of government regeneration initiatives, notes:

> One of the most disturbing features of this experience has been the frequency with which the same areas have to be selected for special treatment; there is overwhelming evidence that earlier programmes were unable to stimulate regeneration on a scale or with sufficient durability to make further special attention unnecessary. Understanding the ingredients of sustainability in the design and implementation of estate and neighbourhood regeneration programmes is therefore of critical importance to both policy makers and practitioners. [Fordham 1995, p. 3]

The report notes a number of structural reasons for concentrations of disadvantage within our communities, and that: 'the impact and consequences of these powerful external forces must necessarily affect the sustainability of local initiatives' (p. 11).

Regeneration programmes are now obliged to include action to build community capacity so that the infrastructures for change which are established during the programme, are enabled to continue and be 'sustained' once the programme has ended. The 1989 Collins Dictionary defines 'sustain' as 'to hold up under; to maintain or prolong; to support physically from below; to provide for or give support to esp. by supplying physical necessities; to keep up the vitality or courage of'. There is now a wealth of practical experience on ways of building this community capacity, which include elements of hard resourcing, as well as skill and knowledge development. These are explored further in Chapter 13 as key elements of building a strategy for community involvement in health. This notion of sustainable infrastructures, which in this form is new to the 1990s, has reinforced the need to see work around community involvement in health as an ongoing, continuous and strategic activity, rather than as a series of *ad hoc* or 'pilot' projects which remain outside the mainstream of an organisation's endeavours. The focus, increasingly, is on change.

However, the change that is required to bring about sustainable regeneration in deprived areas is not only focused on the local community. It is also focused on the policies, practices and services of a range of formal organisations. We have already seen how central government has come to recognise the importance of 'healthy alliances' between the NHS and other organisations and groups as a necessary requirement of improving people's health. Equally it has begun to recognise that the community aspects of regeneration programmes will not be successful without corresponding action at organisational level. The influential Joseph Rowntree Foundation report on creating sustainable regeneration mentioned above recognises this:

> However, problems may also reflect failures in the effectiveness of external services and agencies and their ability to reach disadvantaged communities. If the difficulties of multiply deprived areas are in part a function of the poor design and delivery of main programmes, then sustaining regenerative processes requires external as well as internal change. [Fordham 1995, p. 14]

Therefore sustainable infrastructures need to be built at organisational as well as community levels.

Linking community development with organisation development

While the theory and practice of community development has grown over a number of years within the UK, it has on the whole remained separate from that of organisation development. The latter has more usually taken place within the private sector and business field, and has only recently been applied to the practice of public sector organisations. In the same way that community development is a method of bringing about change within and across communities, so organisation development is a method of bringing about change within the profit world of businesses. Once it began to be used within the public sector worlds of local authorities, health authorities and more latterly, voluntary organisations, its potential for linking in with community development in order to make more effective changes, could be recognised.

We have seen above that there is now a realisation that in order to build sustainable regeneration (which includes a vital element of improving health and well-being), then action within communities and within the services and policies of allied organisations is necessary. This realisation led to the establishment of the CD/OD Network, as a network supported by the Standing Conference on Community Development, in 1994. This is a network of practitioners and academics, who work at both community and organisational levels within different public sector organisations. It aims to explore and promote ways of bringing together work on community and organisation development, in order to bring about more effective change in the empowerment, health and well-being of our communities. The parallels between CD and OD are explored in Chapter 11 on change management.

Notes

1 'Make a Difference': Community Development Consultative Conference, 3–4 December 1996, London, organised by the Standing Conference on Community Development and the Community Development Foundation, and sponsored by the Department of National Heritage.
2 Osborne and Gaebler (1991), *Reinventing Government*. Cited by Trevor Hancock (see note 3).
3 Trevor Hancock, Public Health Consultant, Canada, speaking at the international symposium, 'Health and the Urban Environment: Promoting Good Practice Globally', Manchester, 29–30 June 1994.

4 Why is community involvement in health important now?

Summary

This chapter considers the benefits of community involvement in health to individuals, to communities, to organisations and to society as a whole. It describes the advantages of facilitating the passage from 'passive recipients to active participants' from the perspective of each of those four groups. Brief case studies are described from a wide range of work which has achieved community involvement in health.

All such benefits essentially derive from the nature of the key elements of a community involvement approach to health which have been summarised by Labyrinth in the following list.

Elements of community involvement in a health context:

- Work to actively counter prejudice and discrimination through equal opportunities and positive action.
- Often prioritise work with deprived and disadvantaged groups and communities – be they geographical or communities of interest.
- Make their major focus collective action and change, taking a collective approach to the social causes of ill-health.
- See process, that is, the way of working, as crucial in defining outcomes, so that the process is important in its own right.
- Inter-link not compartmentalise, problems and concerns so a community involvement approach to health encompasses all aspects of people's lives which influence their health potential.
- Encompass a commitment to a holistic approach to health.

- Recognise the central importance of social support and social networks in bringing about change.
- Attempt to facilitate individual and collective action around common needs and concerns, as identified and prioritised by people themselves.
- Are concerned with the opening up of access to information to assist people in making realistic and informed choices and decisions.
- Work to open up professional boundaries and statutory organisations to make them more responsive to people's needs and concerns.

Benefits to individuals

In 1948 the World Health Organization (WHO) Constitution defined health as 'a state of complete physical, mental and social well-being, not merely the absence of disease and infirmity'. This definition has, since then, been adapted and expanded but health is retained by the WHO as a 'holistic' concept. Benefits of community involvement to individuals are more easily seen when such a broad, social definition of health is used, although they can also be seen in a physical, medical context.

At individual level, community involvement in health is important because:

- Interest in and validation of people's experience and views can be health-enhancing in its own right.
- An empowerment approach to involvement challenges apathy and alienation, builds confidence and skills and contributes to a feeling of increased self-esteem and well-being.
- Developing the skills, knowledge, experience and confidence of local people increases their ability to play a greater part in their own health and health care delivery.
- It brings about healthy changes in lifestyle, services or policies which individuals have fought for and which lead directly to individual health benefits.
- It promotes better access for people to health information and resources, greater awareness of an individual's own health needs and those of their community, and of the factors that influence health. It helps people to make realistic and informed decisions about their health.
- Skills learnt through community involvement can be extended and used in other areas of a person's life and expressed in the larger community.

- Individuals can use newly acquired skills and confidence to achieve personal development and material gains which are directly health-enhancing, for instance through access to improved training, education and employment.
- It encourages decisions to be made by people on their own behalf, which are often more realistic and sustainable than those made for them by others.
- It encourages commitment, motivation and shared responsibility.
[Adapted and added to from Smithies 1992]

However, for the individual person, and noting that the theme of this book is the transition of individuals from 'passive recipients' to 'active participants', one of the greatest benefits of community involvement must be the recognition of individuals as 'whole people' rather than as, simply, 'patients' or 'service users'. This is aptly summed up in a poem by Steve Skinner (1997) which appears at the beginning of his book, *Building Community Strengths*:

I'm not just a service user

No I'm not just a service user,
I'm not just a face in the queue,
I'm not just a mum or a member,
I'm a person through and through.

I'm not just the blind or the needy,
Not just one of the deserving few,
So don't give me your charity handouts,
I'm a person through and through.

And I'm not just a wheelchair user,
That others so often see through,
And I'm not just the homeless in doorways,
I'm a person through and through.

I'm not just your client or helper,
Not a vandal or sniffer of glue,
And I'm not the grassroots or just local,
I'm a person through and through.

And I'm not just a single parent,
And my kids aren't a problem to you,
And I'm not just the gypsy they're moving again,
I'm a person through and through.

So I'm not just a service user,
I'm not just a face in the queue,

I'm not just a name or a number,
I'm a person through and through.

So it's time now to drop all your labels,
Start talking both straight and true,
Cos I'm me with my rights, my loves and my fights,
Watch out now cos I'm coming through,
Watch out now cos I'm coming through.

Benefits to communities

People get involved in activities to improve health as individuals, but often that involvement takes a communal form. At individual level someone may get involved through filling in a questionnaire concerning their satisfaction with a particular service, or as an assessment of their health needs. They may act as a carer for an ill person, or as an advocate for a needy individual. They may act in many different ways as a volunteer helper to a person in need. Even at this individual level there are clear benefits to the community as well as to the individual: these acts are an indication of a caring and interested community and if knowledge about them is spread and shared, it can encourage others to get involved in these ways to the greater benefit of all. Volunteering and caring, providing they are backed up by a support system which meets the needs of all those involved, and not just the 'cared for', can be health-enhancing for all.

However, benefits to the community of community involvement in health are more usually seen when that involvement is collectivised and communal. People may get involved in health through many sources, including:

- Social groups.
- Family groups.
- Residents' groups.
- Community groups.
- Trade unions.
- Places of work.
- User groups.
- Self-help groups.
- Community centres and so on.

Their methods of involvement can vary enormously, as described in Part II of this book. They may, for instance, be involved in a community health needs assessment as a group; campaign against health-reducing activities and initiatives, such as campaigns against industrial pollution, or for health-enhancing measures, such as campaigns for pedestrian crossings; set up their own self-help health group to provide support to each other and so on. As communities, people can also be involved in long-term partnerships with other community organisations, and with voluntary and statutory organisations, to improve the health of their local area. Such community initiatives can be *ad hoc*, arising in response to particular circumstances or initiatives, or can be developed and supported strategically, as we describe in Part III of this book. In these cases the benefits of community involvement in health to local communities is increased considerably, as detailed below.

Tackling inequalities in health

Community involvement assists the targeting of disadvantaged or isolated groups, allowing for a shift in focus from traditional priorities. Resources for community involvement enable the setting up of community groups in an area of those who are 'usually excluded' from decision-making processes, for instance youth empowerment groups, a homeless peoples' group, a group of ethnic minority elders, and so on. It is easier, then, for these groups to speak out and have an input into the decision-making processes of other groups and organisations – they are no longer isolated, either as individuals or as marginalised groups. In this sense particular disadvantaged communities are enabled to have their voices heard and health needs met, which is of benefit to those communities; the wider geographical community, of which they are part, also benefits as people within it begin to see the diversity within their own communities as well as its commonalities and to take action to meet their different as well as common needs.

Community involvement, work is often prioritised with deprived and disadvantaged groups and communities, be they geographical or communities of interest. Community development approach, which underpins community involvement, works to counter prejudice and discrimination through creating equal opportunities and positive action.

Building a community infrastructure and network

Community involvement helps the formation of groups, organisations and support structures which provide a resource for many local people and can play an important preventative role, for instance in halting the social decline of an area. Community involvement also recognises the central importance of social support and social networks in bringing about change. For instance, as the community involvement process brings different groups together, it allows people to express their differences but also to discuss and take action on the issues they share. Such shared discussion across communities helps people to see that problems and concerns are interlinked and not compartmentalised into employment, education, housing or health problems – action on many fronts is necessary to improve health.

Community involvement, if adequately resourced, also leads to the development of strong community-controlled institutions on both a geographic and interest-group basis, and includes hard resources/assets such as buildings and equipment, controlled by the community. This is a particularly strong feature of the government-initiated regeneration projects and community partnerships. Once within the control of the community, such assets can then be used by a range of new groups, providing that such community control is open and inclusive.

Improved and appropriate services

Through their own involvement, communities can exert greater influence over health policies and the allocation of resources. They can press for and achieve improved services, or new services which more appropriately meet their needs. This can take the form of:

- Improvements in existing services, for instance improved housing, or improved waiting areas in hospitals.
- New services run by the authorities, for instance a new health centre or 'one-stop shop'.
- New community-run services, for instance a new community centre, or a children's playscheme.
- Ongoing community involvement in the management or decision-making processes of services so that changes can be monitored and new needs fed in easily.
- Greater take-up of services by members of the community, particularly disadvantaged communities, through recognition of their needs and changes to meet those needs.

Improved quality of the environment

The health of communities benefits from community involvement when it leads to direct improvements in the environment. For instance, many participatory health needs assessments have revealed issues of pollution, street cleaning, derelict and dirty buildings, dumping, graffiti, and so on.[1] Local residents are also usually very concerned about the outside appearance of their area, such as smartness of housing, cleanliness of all public areas, facilities for children and older people. In many cases action to tackle these issues has followed. This has ranged from action by the local community (such as clean-up days), to action by local businesses (to tidy their premises), to action by the local authority (to clear up areas of rubbish dumping).

Other aspects of the environment have also been improved following community pressure, for instance improved playspace for children, and improved parks and green areas. The community have also become actively involved in movements to increase safety and reduce crime in their areas and have often worked with the police and other agencies to achieve these ends.

Benefits to organisations

Organisations which have a role to play in promoting good health and improving the population's health, achieve real gains for themselves as well as for their clients or users when they pro-actively seek to increase community involvement in health. These benefits lie within the areas of professional infrastructure, organisation development, targeting and take-up of services, and a shift in balance of resources.

An effective professional infrastructure

Statutory bodies, such as health and local authorities, NHS trusts and Primary Care Groups, are increasingly required by central government to work in 'partnership' with each other, that is, to collaborate in planning and delivering services, and to share visions and missions. We have discussed elsewhere in Part I the growing recognition of the importance of 'healthy alliances' in achieving health gain. A key aspect of this work is the impetus given to professionals within and between agencies to work together. This is not a new approach (some professionals have worked across agency boundaries for many years). What is new is the emphasis given by central government to joint working, and that this emphasis is framed within a strategic context; *ad hoc* responses to joint working are not enough.

We have seen above how a community emphasis on health invites connections to be made between different issues, different services and thus different organisations; health needs to co-operate with housing, education, leisure and so on. It is not surprising that measures to promote community involvement in health are often combined with measures to build inter-agency professional infrastructures. North Staffordshire Health Authority, for instance, funds and supports a number of neighbourhood forums within its area, which are essentially regular meetings of a range of professionals to debate issues of joint concern and to take action within the community to tackle these issues (see the Appendix for the address of the Healthy Alliance Team). Such networking structures can then be used to meet the needs for co-operation between and within a number of different agencies. They also give recognition to and strengthen the need to ensure that the performance of professionals reflects values of empowerment.

A catalyst for organisation development and change

We have described elsewhere the role of organisation development in facilitating community involvement in health and in bringing about the changes within organisations that community involvement requires. When community involvement is seen as something which is only concerned with action at community level (for example, setting up self-help groups, or taking individual responsibility for health) then the implications for wider organisations are limited. With the growing emphasis on the strategic implications of community involvement, organisation development becomes a clear requirement. Communities, once they become empowered and accustomed to having a voice on health issues, begin to look for ways in which they can influence the decisions of those organisations which have a major effect on their lives and their health. In order for such partnerships between communities and organisations to work effectively, not only does the community need to develop new knowledge, skills and understanding, but so do members of those organisations, at all levels.

Seminars attended by senior health purchasers in 1993 identified a range of skills and knowledge which would be needed by members of purchasing organisations in order to take forward community involvement in health purchasing (Labyrinth 1993b). These were:

● Knowledge.
   – what is already going on in NHS and other sectors re community involvement;
   – awareness of local voluntary sector;
   – audit of organisation development needs; and
   – audit of organisational training needs.
● Skills.
   – visioning for the future;
   – changing the organisational culture;
   – changing issues into policy, for example equal opportunities;

- participatory management style;
- internal communication (also a mechanism);
- team building;
- public relations;
- managing change;
- alliance building;
- conflict management; and
- feedback techniques (to local people).

● Attitudes.

- commitment across whole organisation;
- ownership across whole organisation;
- opening up the organisation to wider influence;
- equal opportunities;
- corporate identity;
- encouragement and promotion of innovation; and
- flexible working practices.

The need for organisation development becomes obvious within such a context. Community involvement, then, becomes a catalyst which helps organisations re-examine their purpose, cultures, systems and mechanisms and thus improve their functioning at all levels and on all issues. In particular, when an organisation has a history of promoting community involvement, it is able to provide evidence that its power structures as well as its performance are genuinely open to influence from the outside.

Effective take-up and targeting of services

Organisations are continually seeking to improve the take-up of their services; a quantitative increase in use is a requirement imposed on all health authority contracts with health providers, by the Department of Health through the regional NHS Executives. Similarly some of the targets contained within the Department of Health's health strategy for England, *The Health of the Nation* (1993), were concerned with increased use of health services.

Linked to this is the issue of targeting. Typically community development approaches to health 'reach the parts [of the population] that other [approaches] do not reach'. Community development is essentially about involving people, especially the most disadvantaged, in issues that are important to them. There are many examples throughout the UK where, with the use of skilled, enabling community development techniques, different disadvantaged communities have become more involved in their own health. This has made it easier for health organisations to access those communities, to reach out to them and involve them in their own planning and delivery mechanisms. The case studies at the end of this chapter describe some of the different communities which health organisations have been able to target successfully through the use of community development approaches.

Targeting, too, is one way in which an organisation can demonstrate commitment to its equal opportunities policy and to putting into practice the principle of 'reducing health inequalities', a key aspect of the World Health Organization's 'Health For All' agenda.

At the same time, the nature of the health disadvantages experienced by different communities has meant that a 'quick fix' response by organisations has been ineffective and unsustainable. Ongoing involvement of particular communities has required ongoing commitment from organisations. Again this has forced organisations to critically examine their usual practices and mechanisms and has, in turn, strengthened the case for organisation development and change described above.

An emphasis on prevention

Ultimately and logically a new emphasis on involving the community in health should lead to a shift in the balance of resources, with gradually more proportionately being spent on prevention of ill health and promotion of good health, and a lower proportion on illness and care. That is, health purchasers will be spending an increasing proportion of their budget on purchasing health promotion and illness prevention services. Local Voices (NHSME 1993) promoted the idea that the commissioning role of health authorities should include improving the health of their local populations, not simply commissioning health care services. This has been further strengthened by the 1998 NHS White Paper which requires health authorities to co-ordinate the development and implementation of Health Improvement Programmes. Increasingly local government spending, too, is concerned with activities which promote health and well-being. Simply, this shift in balance is implied because communities bring with them a wider agenda on health, which is as much concerned with tackling social as with medical influences.

Systematic and comprehensive policies

A strategic approach to community involvement in health helps to build structures and mechanisms for consultation and participation at all levels – individual, group, community and agency-wide ('infrastructure'). This means that the input of 'local voices' to organisational decision making is not *ad hoc* and random, but is systematic and comprehensive. If a strategic approach is followed (see, for instance, Chapter 13) then an organisation can be assured that the community input it is receiving is representative, and the discussions and decision making it is engaged in with communities is realistic and sustainable. A full range of user, carer and community groups, and of representative forums for such groups, can play a considerable role as effective mechanisms of consultation on a range of policy issues.

The benefit to organisations is the establishment of an effective system of two-way communication of new ideas, issues and needs between the community and policy makers, whether they originate at community or at organisational levels.

Benefits to society

Community involvement in health will benefit society as a whole:

- It provides a mechanism to tackle variations and inequalities in health and so create a more balanced society in health terms.
- It will help to ensure that changes in planning, providing and monitoring a whole range of health promotion and health care services are sustainable, for the benefit of all, as the ownership and commitment will be shared with the general public as well as with professionals and organisations.
- Through community involvement a number of participatory mechanisms are set up within and between communities, and between communities and wider organisations including local councils, health authorities and trusts, and voluntary organisations; this broadens and strengthens our democracies.
- Community involvement contributes to long-term community education, which helps to build the knowledge and confidence necessary for democracy. This complements the participatory mechanisms described above and helps to ensure they work effectively.
- It plays a crucial role in delivering the 'Health For All' envisaged by the World Health Organization and its member states. This is described in detail below.

Health For All

The future health and well-being of the world's children, of the coming generations, through much better chances of:

- being born healthy;
- to parents who want them;
- who have the time, means and skills to care for them;
- being educated in societies that endorse the basic values of healthy living and free choice, individually exercised;
- being provided with basic requirements for health;
- effectively protected against disease and accidents;
- equal opportunity of living in a stimulating environment;
- social interaction;
- free from the risk of war;
- full opportunities for playing satisfying economic and social roles;
- equal opportunity of growing in a society that supports the maintenance of capabilities;
- provides for secure, purposeful retirement;
- offers care when needed; and
- allows dying with dignity. [Taken from the World Health Organization 1988]

Case Study: 'Look After Yourself' activities in Airedale, West Yorkshire

The health promotion programme for adults, 'Look After Your Heart; Look After Yourself', was developed from a 1978 Health Education Council health and fitness campaign. In 1987 the re-designated Health Education Authority (HEA) subsumed the original LAY programme under a new Coronary Heart Disease information and prevention programme. The HEA provided a national certificated tutor training and staff development structure but programme provision was managed locally.

Airedale Health Authority managed its LAY programme through the Health Promotion Unit in Bradford. This unit decided to adopt a community development approach to the programme because they were particularly concerned to use it to reach individuals and groups in greatest health need, and put a particular emphasis on empowerment and raising self-esteem. This unit had a history of using community development in its approach to health promotion and so developed the LAY programme along community development lines. In 1993 Airedale Health Authority decided to review the values and benefits of the LAY programme locally and the information below is obtained from that review. (Following the dissolution of what was Airedale Health Authority at the end of November 1992, the geographical area covered by this report now lies within the jurisdiction of Bradford Health Authority and North Yorkshire Health Authority.)

The review analysed the views of key staff in health promotion, LAY tutors and course participants. Part of the summary stated:

> LAY in Bradford and Airedale is successful in reaching and involving community groups and population groups who are most in need of this service.
>
> It is successful in bringing about change in individual behaviour to improve health. The group process is essential to this success because it provides the support necessary for people to make and maintain that change.
>
> Its success derives from giving equal weight to the use of empowerment and community development approaches, as to the essential LAY elements of exercise, relaxation and health topics. [Labyrinth 1993c, p. 5]

Benefits to individual participants

During the period of study the LAY classes included the following priority groups. Thirty-two per cent involved elderly people, 36 per cent were women only (these were described as local women, young mothers or Asian women), 18 per cent were specifically for the Asian community, 14 per cent were for people from specific health groups (stroke rehabilitation, coronary rehabilitation, mental illness, people with disabilities) and 11 per cent for colleagues (in a school or hospital). Only 7 per cent were described as being for a 'cross section' of people. They listed the benefits to them as improved fitness, increased knowledge and awareness of health, reduction in stress, reduction in smoking and consumption of fat, salt and sugar, personal well-being, confidence to exercise, gains in confidence and self-esteem, social skills and socialisation, sharing and overcoming similar difficulties, providing time for themselves, recognising their own health and what to do about it.

Benefits for communities

In this context participants described the spread and sharing of information to the wider community, putting health on the local agenda, seeing influences on health as environmental rather than simply individual, support and cohesion, lobbying for improved facilities for a healthier life, greater knowledge and demystification of health, tackling inequalities in health through targeting, shared and co-operative ventures, socialising and having fun and setting up new groups such as a swimming club.

Benefits for the health service

People felt that the health service benefited from LAY primarily through prevention and the reduction in the number of people who needed community or hospital services. People reported, for instance, lowered blood pressure and increased mobility of stroke survivors. They felt there would be less drain on NHS resources through improved health and fitness, and that pressure is taken off NHS staff to discuss health issues in depth, when patients can be referred to `LAY classes. They also felt that LAY classes represented good public relations for the NHS, giving a message that 'needy' groups are not forgotten and that local people are not only being listened to but also educated in how to act on useful health advice. They felt that with increased self-confidence they were able to ask more assertively for the sort of health service or treatment that they wanted.

The review also found that this community development approach to LAY helped build intersectoral working and healthy alliances. Tutors were recruited from all sectors, only minimally from the health service. Venues were provided by a range of organisations, often free of charge. Crèches and other back-up services were provided by different agencies to support the classes.

Case Study: Ince Community Health Project

The Ince Community Health Project began its life in January 1993 following a successful application for Urban Aid. It was set up jointly by the Environmental Health Department of the Metropolitan Borough of Wigan, and the Public Health and Health Promotion Department of Wigan (now Wigan and Bolton) Health Authority. Its purpose was to enable the community of Ince to develop local initiatives to improve their health and well-being. Funded for three years, the project adopted a community development approach to health from the beginning. An outside evaluation of the project took place between September and December 1995 and this case study draws on that evaluation report (Labyrinth 1995a).

The evaluation was carried out in a participatory way, using a mixture of individual and group interviews, observation, and analysis of relevant written material and records. Those interviewed included local residents and members of groups, project workers, management group members, service managers and purchasers from key agencies, and other key individuals within the community, voluntary sector, local authority and health authority.

Benefits to individuals

- Skill development – Participants experienced increased self-confidence through involvement in groups set up or facilitated by the project, and in the training provided by the project or to which they were referred from the project.
- Improved health – This was mentioned by a group of elderly people supported by the project, a new MIND group set up through the project, a Gingerbread group for single parents set up by the project and a new Residents' Association facilitated by the project. People mentioned their improved mental health, stimulation, increased fitness. They mentioned action to tidy up the estate, get housing repairs done quicker, get the environment cleaned up, support a family with a member with Alzheimer's disease and so on, which had resulted from the project's work.

Benefits to community groups

- Access and dialogue with local agencies.
- Work with a broad range of groups.
- Access to community grants.
- Practical help to set up and maintain groups.

Benefits to the community of Ince

- Information access point – This became an increasingly useful focus for the project as other services left the area.
- Reaching the uninvolved – The project drew in those who do not normally get involved.
- Improving morale – An opportunity to show that the community and the project do care.

Benefits to service providers and purchasers

- Joint working with other agencies – The project provided a networking focus for all agencies who had workers in the area and undertook joint projects with them, for example in Heart Health, Sports and Leisure.
- Information on community-led services – The project worked with local people to produce a directory of services and groups in the area.
- The gap was bridged between NHS structures and users.
- Locality commissioning – It was felt that the community infrastructure established in Ince through the work of the project meant there

was potential regarding local involvement in the locality advisory group, although this had not yet been taken up by the health authority.

● A model for others to use – The local Council for Voluntary Service had used the work of the project to take forward good practice elsewhere.

Case Study: Hutson Street Health Project (Bradford)

Hutson Street Health Project is a community development health project working with residents in a particular part of Bradford, West Yorkshire. It is part of the Hutson Street Neighbourhood Project, an inter-agency project between the health authority, social services and the Church. The information in this case study is taken from an evaluation carried out in 1996 (Kilminster 1996).

The aims and objectives of the project are to carry out direct health work with individuals and groups in the community; facilitate and empower the local community to become involved in health and carer issues; act as a bridge between the local community and health professionals; contribute a health perspective to environmental/regeneration work in the area, and undertake training in community development approaches with other professionals. The evaluation found that the evidence collected clearly demonstrated that the project was meeting all of its stated aims and objectives.

Effects of the project for local people

The project affects local people's feelings and knowledge about health and their confidence and quality of life. It is a valued resource for both local people and professionals. In their view the project is directly affecting those factors that affect health and is making a direct contribution to improving the health of local people.

Effects of the health project for its partners in the Hutson Street Project

There is a strong consensus that the partnership is beneficial for all its members and results in the whole project being more than the sum of its parts. The presence of the health project enables the integration of work on health issues into the work of the whole project.

Effects of the health project on local agencies

Health is seen as a multi-agency issue by individuals and agencies in this area. The health project enables more intensive multi-agency working and so enables health needs to be addressed in the most effective way in this inner city area where many residents face multiple disadvantage.

Case Study: Old Trafford Ethnic Communities Health Forum

In 1996 Salford and Trafford Health set up a project to enable the ethnic minority communities of Old Trafford to influence the purchasing decisions of the health authority and its contracts with providers. It wanted to do this through training and developing a group of skilled local people to identify local health needs and to feed these into the health authority. It received resources from the NHS Ethnic Minority Health Unit to carry out the project.

The project worked through recruiting a number of representatives from local ethnic minority communities, analysing their training needs, carrying out the training, and supporting them to carry out health needs assessments in their local communities. It is currently at the stage of considering these needs and action necessary to meet them; and considering the specific and wider implications of the work undertaken with community representatives.

The community representatives involved in the training identified the following benefits of their involvement:

- How to represent the views of my community with the health authority.
- Greater awareness of how the health service works.
- Greater awareness of the problems faced by other ethnic groups.
- Information and advice to pass to the community, such as the difference between GP fundholders and non-fundholders, or how to complain.
- Greater awareness of the availability of local health services to pass to others.
- Ability to assess health needs with my local community.
- Recognition of the advocacy role of the local community.

Note

1   See, for instance, any of the reports of participatory needs assessment carried out in different parts of the UK, available from Labyrinth Training & Consultancy.

Part II

Moving from theory into practice

This part describes a number of different models, tools and techniques which can encourage and support community involvement in health. They are designed to help people think about their own practice and implement appropriate activities both within their own organisations and in direct work with local people and communities. The approaches discussed can be used at many levels. For instance, definitions of 'participation' and 'involvement', and tools designed to facilitate the management of change, are both as important at organisational decision-making levels as within community groups. Equally, these models can be used effectively to stimulate collaboration and action at inter-agency levels in building 'healthy alliances'.

Case studies are used to give examples of each model in practice.

5   Key concepts

This chapter defines the concepts used most commonly in work around community involvement in health. It also gives a categorisation of community groups to illustrate the range and different types of community groups that might exist in an area. This should help planners and community health workers uncover the full range of community groups that exist in their area and so decide which parts of the community they want to involve in a piece of work and at what level.

Community

Collins Dictionary defines community as:

- The people living in one locality.
- The locality in which they live.
- A group of people having cultural, religious or other characteristics in common.
- The public society.
- Similarity or agreement; community of interests.
- The smallest unit of local government.

In a community development context, community can be usefully defined as a group of people who share an interest, a neighbourhood, or a common set of circumstances. They may, or may not, acknowledge membership of a particular community.

In community development terms it is important to remember that people define for themselves which communities they feel part of and this cannot be imposed upon them. They may feel they are members of more than one community and there may be differences between those communities; communities are not homogeneous. This is why community development talks of 'communities' rather than 'the community'.

At the same time planners often need a tool to help them to categorise community needs. In this context some recent research carried out by Labyrinth (1993b) has identified four different ways in which health authorities have categorised communities in planning their work. Some authorities use one category, some all four, and others use a mixture:

- Communities of interest, for example black and ethnic minority people, carers, older people.
- Users of services, for example mental health service users, users of maternity services, patients.
- Localities, for example neighbourhoods, patches, estates, villages.
- The general public.

Community capacity building

The definition of capacity building used by Steve Skinner in his book, *Building Community Strengths* (1997, pp. 1–2), is:

> Development work that strengthens the ability of community organisations and groups to build their structures, systems, people and skills so that they are better able to define and achieve their objectives and engage in consultation and planning, manage community projects and take part in partnerships and community enterprises.
>
> It includes aspects of training, organisational and personal development and resource building, organised in a planned and self-conscious manner, reflecting the principles of empowerment and equality.

Community development

In 1948 the United Nations defined community development as: 'A movement to promote better living for the whole community, with active participation and if possible on the initiative of the community, but if this initiative is not forthcoming, by use of techniques for arousing and stimulating it'.

In 1995 the Standing Conference on Community Development published its own definition of community development as the SCCD Charter:

This is the 'touchstone' of SCCD, providing a point of identification and connection for members. The Charter is not a fixed definition but a tool which can help towards a collective understanding of community development values and provides a common starting point.

Community Development is crucially concerned with the issues of powerlessness and disadvantage: as such it should involve all members of society, and offers a practice that is part of a process of social change.

Community Development is about the active involvement of people sharing in the issues which affect their lives. It is a process based on the sharing of power, skills, knowledge, and experience.

Community Development takes place both in neighbourhoods and within communities of interest, as people identify what is relevant to them.

The Community Development process is collective, but the experience of the process enhances the integrity, skills, knowledge and experience, as well as the quality of power, for each individual who is involved.

Community Development seeks to enable individuals and communities to grow and change according to their own needs and priorities, and at their own pace, provided this does not oppress other groups and communities, or damage the environment.

Where Community Development takes place, there are certain principles central to it.

The first priority of a Community Development process is the empowering and enabling of those who are traditionally deprived of power and control over their common affairs. It claims as important the ability of people to act together to influence the social, economic, political and environmental issues which affect them. Community Development aims to encourage sharing, and to create structures which give genuine participation and involvement.

Community Development is about developing the power, skills, knowledge and experience of people as individuals and in groups, thus enabling them to undertake initiatives of their own to combat social, economic, political and environmental problems, and enabling them to fully participate in a truly democratic process.

Community Development must take a lead in confronting the attitudes of individuals and the practices of institutions and society as a whole which discriminate unfairly against black people, women, people with disabilities and different abilities, religious groups, elderly people, lesbians and gay men, and other groups who are disadvantaged in our society. It must also take the lead in countering the destruction of the natural environment on which we all depend.

Community Development is well placed to involve people equally on these issues which affect us all.

Community Development should seek to develop structures which enable the active involvement of people from disadvantaged groups, and in particular people from black and ethnic minority groups. [SCCD, UKACW and FCWTG 1995]

Community development and health (CDH)

Similar principles, values, concepts and words are used when applying a definition of community development to a health context. The definition developed by Healthy Sheffield and used by its partner agencies including Sheffield Health, Sheffield Council and key voluntary and private sector organisations is typical:

> Community Development aims to enable the active involvement of people, especially those most oppressed and marginalised, in issues, decision-making and organisations which affect their health and lives in general.
>
> It can take place at the grass roots, in neighbourhoods or communities of interest and also at an organisational level in policy, planning and service delivery. It is based upon people identifying their own needs and how these can best be met. It involves enabling people to come together to share experience, knowledge and skills; to support their participation and encourage their involvement in influencing policy making and service development on issues which concern them.
>
> Integral to the Community Development approach is a commitment to equal opportunities and confronting inequality and discrimination.
>
> A Community Development approach to health emphasises the holistic nature of health, and a positive approach to health, well-being and its promotion. [Healthy Sheffield Support Team 1993]

Community group

When people acknowledge membership of a shared community they may form a community group by meeting together for a particular purpose. This may be on the basis of locality (for instance, a tenants' or residents' association) or of common interest (for instance, a city-wide pensioners' group). People may come together as a group to focus on a particular issue, such as health or children's play, or with a broader focus on general needs. As a result of forming a group, a network between people in a particular community is formed. Community groups are essentially run and organised by the members within them, rather than by outside people, although outsiders can, through the community development process, play a facilitative role in enabling people to run their own groups.

The categorisation system below was developed by Labyrinth as an aid in identifying the broad range of community groups that might exist in an area and as a tool in carrying out a community audit.

Table 5.1   Community groups: a categorisation

TYPE	NEIGHBOURHOOD e.g. Tenants' Association	INTEREST e.g. Pensioners' Group	USERS e.g. Maternity Services
FOCUS	GENERAL e.g. Community Association	SINGLE e.g. Health Group	
SPREAD	SINGLE COMMUNITY e.g. Young Women's Group	COALITION e.g. Federation of Community Associations	
PURPOSE	SERVICE DELIVERY e.g. Holiday Playscheme	SELF-HELP e.g. Support Group	CAMPAIGN e.g. Changes in Policy

When considering any initiative around community involvement in health it is important to carry out an audit of existing groups. A recent audit within Kirkby on Merseyside discovered a broad range of community groups (Labyrinth 1994a, p. 14). The audit then considered a further categorisation based on relevance to health. It found that some community development groups had health as an explicit overall focus, for instance the Women's Health Project, the Kirkby Drugs Project and the Community Health Forum; other groups had an explicit interest in health along with other interests e.g. the Tower Hill Young Women's Group held some health information sessions. Some groups campaigned on explicit health issues, for instance KAPIT which is campaigning against a medical waste incinerator being built in Kirkby. Other groups were seen by others to undertake activity relevant to health, for instance groups established through the Save the Children Childminder Development Project and focusing on childcare and parenting; while yet others could be seen in a health-promoting light whatever their focus, where community activity is seen as enhancing health and well-being.

Consultation, involvement and participation

It is useful to link these three terms as they are often used interchangeably, whereas in fact they have quite distinct meanings. Collins Dictionary defines these words in the following way:

Consult: To seek advice, to refer to for information
Involve: To include or contain as a necessary part, to have an effect on
Participate: To take part in, to become actively involved in, to share in

Participation has become a byword in many spheres, notably in social planning. It is seen as a crucial element in community work practice. The following diagram may be helpful in considering degrees of participation in specific situations; the lower levels of participation described in this diagram might more appropriately be labelled as consultation.

Empowerment

This can be defined as 'the process of redefining, experiencing and realising one's own power' (Kramarae and Treichler 1985), or as 'a working style which aims to help people achieve their own purpose by increasing their confidence and capacity', as described in David Wilcox's *Guide to Effective Participation* (1994, p. 41).

Infrastructure

A community infrastructure is one of the five key elements of a community involvement strategy described fully in Chapter 13. The development of a community infrastructure is sometimes described as community capacity building. In practice there is great overlap between these two concepts and the structures which go with them, but they are not precisely the same.

Community infrastructure develops from community work and involves helping community and user groups and development workers to network with each other, to enable them to learn from each other and exchange

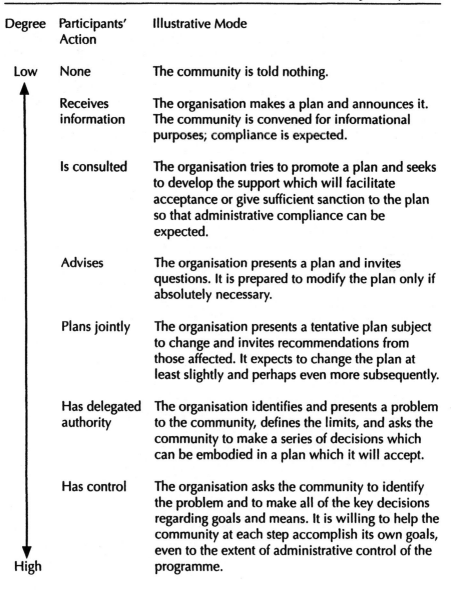

Degree	Participants' Action	Illustrative Mode
Low	None	The community is told nothing.
	Receives information	The organisation makes a plan and announces it. The community is convened for informational purposes; compliance is expected.
	Is consulted	The organisation tries to promote a plan and seeks to develop the support which will facilitate acceptance or give sufficient sanction to the plan so that administrative compliance can be expected.
	Advises	The organisation presents a plan and invites questions. It is prepared to modify the plan only if absolutely necessary.
	Plans jointly	The organisation presents a tentative plan subject to change and invites recommendations from those affected. It expects to change the plan at least slightly and perhaps even more subsequently.
	Has delegated authority	The organisation identifies and presents a problem to the community, defines the limits, and asks the community to make a series of decisions which can be embodied in a plan which it will accept.
High	Has control	The organisation asks the community to identify the problem and to make all of the key decisions regarding goals and means. It is willing to help the community at each step accomplish its own goals, even to the extent of administrative control of the programme.

Figure 5.1 The 'Ladder of Participation'

information and support, so that they can move forward collectively. Participants learn from each other's successes and mistakes so that they do not have to 'reinvent the wheel'. It means that views from a number of different groups and communities can be gathered and brought together.

Examples of activities and structures which are part of a community infrastructure include area/district-wide umbrella forums, such as a Community Health Forum, a Black Health Forum, a Federation of Community Organisations, or a Network of Tenants Associations; accessible centralised information resources which all groups can use, such as a general community resource centre; funding and provision of district/area-wide training opportunities; workshops and conferences on particular community issues, and newsletters or information sheets to which different community groups and organisations contribute (Brager and Specht 1973, p. 39). Clearly these examples, when used in a health context, would have an explicit health focus.

Organisation development

Organisation development within a community involvement and health context aims to improve the effectiveness of the organisation through encouraging participation and responding to the needs and ideas from local communities and users of services. It involves creating an organisational environment which is open, has a long-term outlook, and which develops a strategy for effective change management in a participatory way. It means addressing issues of power and organisational culture, and putting in place systems and structures that are publicly accountable and able to respond to new information, priorities and needs. As such, it is one of the five key elements of a community involvement in health strategy described fully in Chapter 13.[1]

Examples of activities which can be carried out under an organisation development umbrella in this connection include: establishing organisational policy and aims for community involvement; developing an equal opportunities statement of intent, policy, practice guidelines and targets; setting community involvement objectives and targets for each part of the organisation; creating an organisational culture that encourages and enables participation and empowerment; providing managers with training in community involvement and managing change, and reviewing organisation structures and systems.

Organisation development more widely focuses on harnessing the human energy within a group/organisation by realising the full potential of the people within the group/organisation. It assists the effectiveness, capabilities and adaptability of the group/organisation by improving the processes by which people get things done and the relationships between people and groups within the group/organisation.

Organisation development tries to combine group/organisational process with group/organisational structures to meet complementary objectives of human fulfilment and task accomplishment.

Organisation development draws on both the behavioural sciences and the specific business and environmental issues relating to a group/organisation. In practice organisation development intervention takes place at a number of different levels: individual, group, inter-group, and organisation/department-wide; there is often intervention happening at several different levels at the same time.

Sustainability

This word has crept recently into the community development literature from at least two directions. First there is now a clear government requirement that funding bids to the regeneration programmes (many of which incorporate community involvement and partnerships as key elements) illustrate 'sustainability' of programmes and outcomes. Second there is the prominence of the notion of 'sustainable development' in the still-influential 1987 report of the World Commission on Environment and Development, *Our Common Future: From One Earth to One World*. In subsequent linked reports the core meaning of sustainable development embodies a central concern for the health of human societies and the natural environment in the present and the future (Gamble and Weil 1997).

In a context of community involvement in health it is useful to refer to the definition of 'sustain' in Collins Dictionary:

To hold up under; to withstand; to undergo; suffer; to maintain or prolong; to support physically from below; to provide for or give support to, especially by supplying necessities; to keep up the vitality or courage of; to uphold or affirm the justice or validity of; to establish the truth of; confirm.

This seems to indicate that sustainable community involvement in health would require support from a number of different directions (or agencies) and so relates neatly to the mechanisms of community involvement described elsewhere in this book.

Note

1 'Five Key Elements of a Community Involvement Health Strategy', Labyrinth Training and Consultancy handout.

6 Building community action on health

Summary

This chapter describes the main elements of community work and the role it plays in building community action. It begins by discussing community work, its purpose, roles and functions. It then moves on to the principles of community work within a health context and describes in detail the community work process. The chapter describes the 'collective action cycle', one of the basic models developed through community work. This model explores the process through which the experience of individuals (in this case related to health and well-being) is brought together and then shared, collectivised, reflected upon and analysed so that the resultant action on health taken by communities is rooted in their day-to-day lived experiences. The use of this model is key in ensuring that community action on health is sustainable, because it is based on community ownership of their experiences, and brings about their commitment to taking thoughtful action to implement change in their health and well-being. In this way the 'collective action cycle' is a fundamental building block and process in developing community action on health.

Examples are given of the way this model can be used at community level, partnership level (between communities and organisations in joint planning groups) and at top decision-making levels within organisations.

Community work

We have seen in Part I that community development approaches have played a key role in the history and current practice of community involvement in health. Community work is in turn one of the key elements of community development and it is this element which we will explore here.

Community work is essentially the process through which communities are enabled to come together to discuss issues which they see as important to them, and to take action to deal with those issues. Thus community workers are people who play a leading role in structuring and facilitating this process. They may be unpaid members of the community, who are particularly skilled or experienced in working with others to build community action; or they might be paid employees with a job brief which focuses on community work. In this case their employers might be a community or voluntary organisation, or a statutory body such as a local authority, health authority or health trust. Increasingly, community workers are employed by partnership groups which are alliances between a number of organisations, such as a regeneration partnership or a 'Health For All' partnership.

A recent functional analysis of the essential purposes, roles and skills of community work, carried out by the Federation of Community Work Training Groups (1994) found that a key purpose was to: 'Create opportunities for diverse communities collectively to identify needs and rights, clarify objectives and take action to meet these within a developmental framework which respects the needs and rights of different communities in society' (FCWTG 1994 p. 19). They identified at least six key roles for community work:

- Engage with the community and establish agreement for involvement.
- Enable people to work and learn together effectively.
- Enable people to identify and prioritise needs, opportunities and rights and plan collective action.
- Enable people to implement and review collective action.
- Provide organisational support to community activities.
- Manage own work to achieve community and organisational objectives.

It is important that these roles of community work are carried out according to principles of effective working.

Principles of community work and community health work

Community work is not a profession which lays down a sole route of entry or has established a rigid set of principles and practices which all must adopt. It has, rather, sought to ensure that all those with an enthusiasm for building community action are encouraged and supported to take such actions and to enable others to do so. As a result, no one set of agreed principles exists. However, all organisations which are formally concerned with promoting community work, within or without a health context, have established their own set of principles and practices and there is much common agreement. Some of these are listed below.

The Federation of Community Work Training Groups, a nationally recognised body within the community work training and education field, and supported through a core grant from national government (currently from the Department of National Heritage), notes that there are a number of underpinning values required for competent community work practice: 'Competence in the dynamic process of community work requires understanding, integration and practical application of values in the community work relationship, demonstrating a commitment to social justice'. For them this means:

- Being committed to working with groups and communities to enable them to collectively improve or enhance equality of access to the following, for enduring benefit to the group or community:
  - the political and policy-making processes;
  - knowledge and information;
  - decision making;
  - choices;
  - resources; and
  - opportunities for development and enjoyment.

- Recognising and stimulating the expertise, skills, knowledge and creative ideas that exist in the community, and sharing them in a developmental and inter-active way.
- Believing in and respecting the rights, value, diversity and dignity of individuals, groups and communities.
- Practising in a way that challenges inequality, oppression, prejudice and discrimination.
- Ensuring that all activities are consistent with participatory democracy and progressive development.

- Agreeing with groups and communities the mutual obligations involved in community work, action and development, whilst building confidence, trust and autonomy.
- Respecting the rights of groups and communities to define their own problems, issues, interests and goals, and to prioritise action.
- Offering one's self as a positive resource, showing commitment to these values [FCWTG 1994, p. 26].

Other organisations have considered the principles of building community action within an explicit health context. The West Yorkshire Community Health Training Project (1990, unpublished), during its three years of existence between 1987 and 1990, wrote the following brief for community health work. They noted that a community work approach to health entails:

- Increasing the ability of people to work together.
- Developing the skills, knowledge, experience and confidence of local people to play a greater part in their own health and health care delivery.
- Trying to change power structures in order to promote the needs of those groups who are discriminated against and to respond to the effects of discrimination of those groups.

Generally, the project argued, the main features of community health work involve:

- Promoting a positive view of health.
- Taking a collective approach to the social causes of ill health.
- Promoting better access for people to health information and resources.
- Promoting increased self-confidence to enable people to take greater control over their own health.
- Promoting positive changes in the relationship between health workers and local people.
- Enabling greater public influence over health policies and the allocation of resources.
- Reducing inequalities in health by confronting the practices of institutions which discriminate against black people, ethnic minority people, unemployed people, women, older people and other groups; and responding to the effects of discrimination and disadvantage on those groups.

Collective action cycle

The 'collective action cycle' is the most basic process of community work. It describes how it is possible to build collective action and commitment to change, in the area of community health.

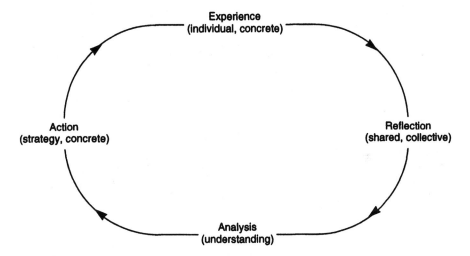

Figure 6.1   The collective action cycle

In its simplest form, a community health worker can initiate and facilitate the collective action cycle in the following way. Often, though, the process may be much more involved and detailed, whilst sticking to this simple form. In all cases it is the rooting of discussion and action in lived experience which is important, and a community worker or community health worker needs the skills to facilitate and structure this:

- Experience – The community health worker creates opportunities for individuals to come together to talk about their personal experiences of particular issues that are important to them, for example health, and facilitates sharing.
- Reflection – The community health worker structures the situation so that the individuals are enabled to listen to each other and make connections between their experiences. She or he asks questions to help pull out similarities and differences.
- Analysis – The community health worker asks lots of 'why' questions so that the group can come to a shared analysis of the issues they are

discussing. She or he may offer relevant information from elsewhere, to help their analysis, if relevant, but always placing it against the experience of those involved.

- Action – The community health worker helps the group to brainstorm possible action they could take to deal with the issue, and to decide which of those they will follow. It might be action involving only themselves ('self-help'); it might involve communicating with other groups and agencies; it might involve an extensive action plan.

Once the action has started, the worker helps the group to reflect on and analyse its success and to agree further action if necessary; in this way they are taken through the cycle again.

The use of this model is key in bringing about the empowerment of those involved. This is because central to it is the validation of people's experiences, skills and knowledge – they are the main focus. Yet it is also a developmental process which enables individuals, groups and communities to move forward and bring about change, within their own lives and in the world around them. It allows for the input of outside information, but the role of the community worker or community health worker is to help that information become relevant to the group by testing it against their own experience. The case studies below describe the use of this process at three levels: community level, partnership level and organisational level.

Case Study: Collective action on health at community level

Hutson Street Health Project in Bradford, West Yorkshire, covers an inner-city area which is considered 'deprived' within the city as a whole. The project employs a community health worker with funding from the local and health authorities on a joint finance basis. The project was set up in 1991 and works on community health in a number of different and interconnecting ways, through establishing a number of different activities, groups and networks. We are concerned here with the process followed by the worker in building collective community action on health among the residents of the local area, rather than with the full range of the worker's activities.

A recent and independent evaluation (Kilminster 1996) confirmed that word of mouth was very important in attracting new users to the project; some came in 'off the street' to see what was happening, others had come for individual advice initially, some had seen publicity material. Once in the project, local people are encouraged to have confidence and trust in the project. The evaluation showed that local people unanimously felt that their confidence and well-being had increased through the project and that their health had improved.

Through such contacts with local people, the worker has set up a number of group activities over the years. At the time of the evaluation (August 1996) these included three groups specifically focusing on health:

- The girls' group meet weekly, they cook a meal together if they are remaining at the centre and undertake a wide variety of activities as well as having a number of discussions.
- The weekly LAY (Look After Yourself) class covers the three areas of exercise, relaxation and discussion of health topics. At each weekly meeting the proportion of time spent on each area varies according to the interests and needs of the group members. There is a crèche.
- The 'cooking for life' group meets weekly and each member prepares and cooks a meal to take home. The aim is to develop skills, confi-· dence and knowledge around cooking and healthy eating and to enable members to try new kinds of foods. There is a crèche.

There are a number of other groups, such as the Credit Union and play-group which have health project involvement. There is also a two-week summer playscheme for children aged 5–12 organised by local people. The worker also plays a key role in working with the management committee so that local residents are enabled to play a full and equal part in its meetings.

The choice of which groups to set up and which issues to discuss are based on the expressed needs of local people. The sympathetic listening and facilitating role of the worker, as well as the presence of support activities such as the crèche, are key in enabling discussion to move on from sharing individual experiences to collective reflection and analysis, and then on to a group decision about activities and action.

The evaluation of the health project showed how effective such an approach was in improving the health of participants. It included an assessment by users of the project of whether they thought their participation in the project affected health-related factors such as regular exercise, smoking, depression, going to a GP, knowledge about health, etc. As the evaluation states: 'The results ... clearly show that the project users consider that the project has a strong positive affect on the factors that influence their health' (Kilminster 1996, p. 7).

Case Study: Collective action on health at partnership level

There are many examples of 'joint planning groups' where 'joint' refers to a coming together of large and often statutory organisations, such as social services departments and health authorities (sometimes with the presence of a voluntary organisation), with no community involvement. If such involvement is sought, it is often confined to one or two 'user' representatives who feel that their involvement is token, with the 'real' decisions taken by others. However, there are examples of joint planning groups where local people are given an equal voice and role to representatives from statutory and voluntary organisations. In these cases the 'collective action cycle' can usually be seen in the processes followed by such groups.

· Colburn is a rural area in North Yorkshire, where health statistics indicate a lower level of health compared to other areas in the same authority. The Colburn Community Health Forum was set up in 1994 on the initiative of North Yorkshire Health Authority and with the involvement of local residents and local agencies. This initiative grew out of a review into how local people in Colburn could become more involved in decisions affecting their health, and how different agencies could work together more effectively to meet the needs of people in Colburn. The review was based on interviews with residents from the area and with people from different key agencies (including statutory services such as education and health, voluntary bodies such as the Citizens' Advice Bureau and community groups such as the Community Association). Based on these interviews the review identified:

- Why community participation and inter-agency working are important for Colburn.
- Particular issues that need to be addressed for progress in these areas.
- A possible way forward for Colburn.

Following this review a workshop was held for local residents and representatives from key agencies to explore the setting up of a Community Health Forum which would be effective in enabling the involvement of local people in decisions affecting their health in partnership with key agencies. Twenty-six people attended this workshop of which almost half were local residents (the others were representatives of a variety of statutory and voluntary agencies active in the area). They had read the report of the review, which stimulated and structured discussion. Participants broke into small groups to discuss, note and make proposals for four related areas:

- Purpose, aims and objectives of the new structure.
- Membership and structure.
- Servicing.
- Budget.

Agreement was reached in all four areas. For example, the workshop decided that their aim should be 'the betterment of life and living in Colburn', their purpose 'to identify local needs and problems, to be driven by local voices and to get some action by influence, pressure and joint working'. They would identify their own objectives, initially based on the recommendations of the recent participatory health needs assessment report. They developed a structure which ensured that core membership should include all community groups for Colburn people, all individuals from Colburn who may have an interest, and all agencies covering the area. They established a set of principles for the Forum which included local ownership, equal partnership, a vision for the whole community not just a group, an emphasis on the delivery of action and monitoring of quality, and facilitation of a 'hub and spoke' mechanism, that is, core activities and a range of other activities feeding into this. They went into great detail about the practices of the Forum, its method of working and effective servicing based on its key principles. As a result, the Community Health Forum for Colburn was set up and continues to take action and to develop.[1]

The collective action cycle is set in motion when a new structure is set up in ways which are built on the experience of those involved and so have their ownership of it, as well as being realistic and sustainable. From the review stage to the workshop stage, there was a clear focus on the experiences of those involved. The initial interviews asked people (residents and professionals) about their experiences of community participation and inter-agency working: what were the successes and positive aspects and what were the barriers and difficulties? The workshop provided a forum for collective discussion of the findings of the review, as well as analysis and reflection. The small-group work provided an opportunity for ideas to be generated on action to be taken, so that the action (that is, the setting up of a Community Health Forum) was properly routed in a collective experience. In this instance, how the Forum was set up and how people decided it should run its business, was seen as important as what the Forum then set out to do. It was based on a recognition from the outset that the views of residents in such a Forum was as important as those of the professionals (and vice versa), in making that forum effective and sustainable.

Case Study 7: Collective action on health at organisational level

The NHS and Community Care Act of 1990 set the policy framework for community involvement in health and community care. Whilst this Act was key in sparking off specific initiatives placed centrally within NHS institutions (such as the initiatives on 'local voices', 'patient charters' and 'participatory health needs assessments' which are pursued elsewhere in this book), it was more explicit about the role of community involvement in community care. Although the crucial role of the NHS in community care is recognised, the Act gave the leading role in this respect to local authority social services departments. The Act placed an obligation on the statutory bodies to involve users, carers and voluntary organisations in drawing up and implementing their Community Care Plans. Subsequently a number of government guidelines have stressed that user and carer involvement should become a crucial part of all aspects of community care including commissioning, planning, evaluating and improving services.

This case study looks at user and carer involvement in community care at organisational levels with specific reference to the 'collective action cycle' because, frankly, social services departments have gone further in this regard than health authorities (perhaps because of the more explicit nature of this reference in the Act) and so more examples of community involvement at organisational levels exist.

Since 1990 Barnsley Social Services, along with other departments elsewhere in the country, has developed a number of initiatives concerned with increasing the involvement of users and carers in their own care plans. However, as things developed they realised that a strategic approach to involvement was needed to address gaps and to take the initiative further. In 1995 they commissioned a review of user and carer involvement in Barnsley, a report of interesting practice elsewhere and a report with recommendations for the development of a strategic approach (Labyrinth 1995d,e).

The conclusions of the review included the following:

- Much of the involvement in community care is centred around individual contact and discussion.
- Carers have a greater degree of involvement than users.
- Promoting involvement needs to concentrate on providing information, resources and training.
- There also needs to be formal structures for involvement and a framework of good practice.

In other words, involvement was on the whole confined to individual user and carer input into their own care plans, and was not visible at broader planning or strategic levels where decisions about priorities, resources, principles, methods of working or broader vision were taken.

The recommendations for a way forward were grouped into three categories: demonstrating visible commitment from the top, developing practical methods for action, and providing resources and support for development. In this way action was encouraged at a number of different levels, including action to build community involvement (in this case of users and carers) at organisational decision-making levels. A key recommendation aimed at this level was the setting up of an inter-agency and user/carer steering group. This recommendation states in full that:

Action and information about user and carer involvement in community care needs co-ordinating across agencies and with the community. A joint Steering Group will aid that co-ordination as well as spreading information to all sectors and all levels, as suggested in the review. It is suggested that this Steering Group:

- Comprises members from social services, health, voluntary sector, user groups and carer groups.
- Meets regularly, say monthly, for an initial period of one year.
- Ensures that each representative feeds back to and from their constituent group (such as department or group).
- Is serviced by a named member of staff with strategic as well as developmental skills, at a sufficiently high level within the department and with admin backup.
- Spends an initial period (say the first three months) in agreeing and acting upon an appropriate structure for the group meeting which clearly aids rather than inhibits partnership and involvement, for instance use of jargon, access, notes, style, chair, measures to ensure equal involvement such as 'pairing' between meetings, how to feed back and from their own groups and departments.
- Writes a brief outline strategy for user and carer involvement, building on the work of this review and the December workshop, which is clear about aim and rationale.
- Sets up a subgroup to develop a training strategy in user and carer involvement ... and organises initial courses.

It is important that the Steering Group is given sufficient authority by all relevant agencies and that it feeds formally into the Joint Care Planning Team and the Policy Advisory Groups.

At the end of the first year the Group should review its progress and consider further action, especially at the upper ends of the autonomy/empowerment ladder ... [Labyrinth 1995d]

The above was one of ten recommendations, each one aimed at addressing different aspects and different levels of an overall strategy. This recommendation cannot be taken in isolation when considering a total involvement strategy, but is detailed here because of its focus on organisational decision making.

Following the review, this Steering Group was set up and spent its first year in negotiating the way it should operate as well as in drawing up the next stage of an action plan. It has representation from users and carers as well as from different statutory and voluntary agencies. It continues to focus as much on process as on content. It is informed by the developmental work taking place with different user and carer groups, as well as by outside agency experiences. This in turn follows a practice used in the review (and in various previous departmental consultations) whereby the views and experiences of a number of different individuals and groups were sought. People were interviewed across all sectors (local authority,

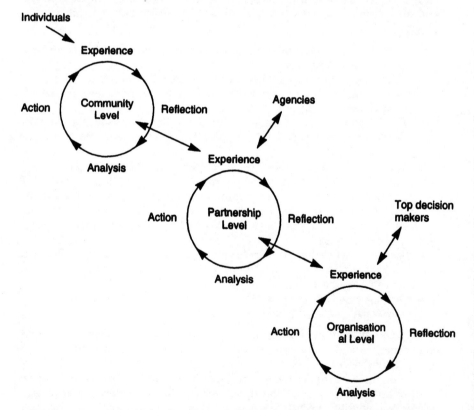

Figure 6.2   Connections between collective action at different levels

health authority, voluntary sector) and at all levels (users, carers, operational workers, managers and planners, top decision makers) regarding their views and experiences of involvement. Following these interviews and a draft report, a workshop was held with all those involved to discuss the findings and firm up the ideas for action into clear recommendations.

In these ways the experiences and knowledge of different individuals, groups and organisations were pooled to develop an action plan and ongoing organisational strategy which could be owned by all those involved.

Note

1 For further information contact Dr Alice Milburn, Health Promotion Advisor, North Yorkshire Health Authority, Sovereign House, Kettlestring Lane, Clifton Moor, York YO3 4XF.

7 Advocacy

Summary

We have seen in Chapter 3 how the advocacy and user involvement movement which has grown up in the last ten years in the UK has enabled many groups who have traditionally been excluded from community activity, and certainly from participation in the affairs of public bodies such as health authorities and trusts, to get and stay involved. This chapter summarises that history but concentrates on the practicalities of advocacy – what it is and how you do it. It begins with listing and describing the various elements of good practice in advocacy. This includes definitions, different types of advocacy with practical examples, and principles and values of advocacy. It explores advocacy in practice, discussing in detail the role of the advocate, the support they need and how to run an advocacy service which is consistent with the key principles and values of advocacy. A checklist of steps to take when setting up an advocacy project follows, along with some ideas for methods of monitoring progress within an advocacy service and who should carry that out. The chapter moves on to describe some of the wider support that is necessary for advocacy to be fully effective and is an important section for organisations who wish to support the development of advocacy, as well as for advocacy services themselves. This section concentrates on a strategic approach to advocacy. The chapter ends with describing some of the benefits of an advocacy approach as perceived by different 'stakeholders' – policy makers and funders, service users, service providers, user advocates, volunteer advocates and carers.

This chapter draws heavily on two documents previously published by Labyrinth. The *Code of Good Practice for Advocacy for Oldham* (Labyrinth

1996a) was commissioned by Oldham Independent Advocacy Steering Group in 1996, while the report *User and Carer Involvement: Some Examples of Interesting Literature and Practice* (Labyrinth 1995e) was commissioned by Barnsley Social Services in 1995.

History

We have already had a brief history of the development of the advocacy and user movements within the UK in Chapter 3. The impetus for this recent growth over the last decade has been twofold. On the one hand 'users' themselves have become more assertive and organised about expressing their voice and have set up their own user or advocacy groups, sometimes with the support of sympathetic voluntary organisations such as MIND (working with mental health service users), or umbrella bodies such as People First (a network of people with learning difficulties). It is interesting that this self-help advocacy movement developed, on the whole, with little input from community development workers or community health workers. Typically, community development workers, with or without a health remit, work with geographic or 'interest' communities (see Chapter 5 on key concepts), rather than with service user groups such as these. And, by the early 1990s, when social services departments and health authorities were beginning to consider advocacy models (see below), the Community Development and Health movement was not organised enough to make practice or theoretical connections with community care initiatives, as discussed in Chapter 2. So the early advocacy movement within the UK was initially heavily influenced by the citizen advocacy movement of the US, which concentrated on individualised one-to-one ways of working, rather than by community development models of working. However, it soon moved to a home-grown model of advocacy, which incorporated citizen advocacy and self-advocacy, and with principles similar to those of community development.[1]

On the other hand, recent legislation has boosted support for advocacy (or the requirement for support) from statutory organisations. The NHS and Community Care Act (1990) places a duty on social services departments and health authorities to consult with users and carers (as well as voluntary organisations) at every level of drawing up, implementing and reviewing policies, strategies and practices in community care. Various sets of policy guidance from the Department of Health following the Act have made the role for advocacy explicit. For example, 'Community Care in the Next Decade and Beyond' (cited in Lovett 1994) states that one of the main objectives of care management is to 'promote individual choice and self determination', while the guidance on Assessment and Care Management recognises the need to inform service users and carers of independent advocacy projects and to be aware of the possible conflicts for service providers acting as advocates on behalf of users of their services. At the same time the mental illness handbook relating to the government's health strategy, 'Health of the Nation', contains many references to advocacy and includes the statement:

> Advocacy is about giving the individual a voice and getting the NHS and Social Services to listen to that voice and to take into account its needs and preferences. In order to ensure that there is no conflict of interests in the representation of service users' views, advocacy therefore needs to be independent of service provision. [Quoted in Lovett 1994, p. 7]

There are many examples of the practical ways in which health or local authorities are supporting advocacy and user involvement. Some have set up User Forums, resourced by development workers; some have set up specific carer or user groups, such as young carers groups, as self-help groups but with outside support. Others have supported advocacy groups within a particular service, or a scheme for independent advocates for individuals. Some have funded or contracted user and/or carer groups and organisations to run and develop their own service. A minority of authorities have begun to see the connections between a community development approach to health and an advocacy approach with service users. They have set up joint health/local authority structures which involve communities and service users and take action on health promotion and commissioning as well as on community care.

What is advocacy?

Advocacy is about people speaking up for or acting on behalf of themselves, possibly with the support of another person/group or 'advocate'. It is also about taking action to get something changed, in order to take more control over our lives. It is about empowering ourselves and others. Taking control can happen at different levels and advocacy has a role to play in all of these:

- Everyday decisions.
- Life-changing decisions.
- Choice over services.
- Control over services.

- Political influence.

Types of advocacy

There are several types of advocacy which operate in different ways. Each is described below, with an example of how they are applied in practice within Oldham in Lancashire, to illustrate the breadth that is possible within one geographic area.

Citizen advocacy

Citizen advocacy is a one-to-one long-term partnership between a service user and a 'citizen' who is acting as a volunteer. The volunteer helps the person to speak up for themselves or speaks for them as appropriate. The volunteers are usually recruited and supported through a paid co-ordinator. Where the relationship is short-term it may be described as *crisis advocacy*.

Within Oldham, there is a specific citizen advocacy scheme, OPAL (Oldham People's Advocacy and Leisure), which provides volunteer advocates for people with learning disabilities, who are supported by a paid co-ordinator. She also meets regularly with each person/volunteer partnership to see how/if the needs of the partner are being met. OPAL co-ordinators have also established 'Advocate associates' who can be called on for specific help. Currently they include a doctor, funeral director, insurance provider, solicitor, accountant and educationalist.

Peer advocacy

Peer advocacy involves one-to-one support by a service user, past or present, to help another to express and fulfil their wishes.

Within Oldham, members of the Oldham Self-Advocacy Group (see below) often act as peer advocates and speak up on behalf of someone else who has contacted the group and requested this help. Group members feel that the self-confidence they have developed through being part of the group, along with their own personal experiences of mental health and mental health services, helps them to be peer advocates. They can stand alongside a person rather than trying to take over.

Self-advocacy

Self-advocacy takes place when groups of people get together to speak out collectively about joint concerns. It can also apply to individuals who speak out for themselves.

Within Oldham, there are a number of examples of self-advocacy, including the Oldham Self-Advocacy Group. This is a group for people who use the mental health services and have formed a committee to ensure that their views are taken into account. They have, for instance, made representation to the Joint Advisory Group and a number of other services-led groups or committees.

Legal advocacy

Legal advocacy is represented by legally qualified advocates, usually solicitors or barristers.

Within Oldham, organisations offering this type of support include the Citizens Advice Bureau, which has a rota of solicitors working with them, and Oldham Law Centre. The Law Centre concentrates on advocating for people on housing, employment and immigration issues. Their Asian Women's Rights Worker can help in some cases.

Professional advocacy

Professional advocacy occurs when a paid worker represents the interests of a person but is independent of the organisation or service to which they are advocating.

Within Oldham, there are a number of examples of professional advocacy. For instance the Community Health Council has a formal and statutory role to monitor health services on behalf of the general public. They are a 'watchdog' and represent individuals who have a complaint against any of the health services. This can involve letter writing, accompanying complainants to an interview or representing them at a formal complaints procedure. The Indian Association employs advice workers who undertake advocacy around a variety of issues – immigration, social security, social and health services. They help the individual to speak up, or will speak up on the individual's behalf, with other individuals or services.

Staff advocacy

Staff advocacy takes place when service staff speak up for individual service users. It is different from professional advocacy because it may involve a conflict of interest: the member of staff is often paid by the organisation they are taking issue with on behalf of the user. Therefore it is more appropriately called *representation* rather than advocacy.

Within Oldham, social workers, nurses and other service staff often represent their clients in this way. For instance staff at Foxdenton School for children with special needs see themselves as playing an advocacy role by helping children and parents articulate their wishes, supporting them in actions they want to take themselves and acting on their behalf to secure a better deal for them. This is done individually but also through surveys and questionnaires, so that children and parents can feed in their thoughts about ways of improving existing services.

Service staff generally also play a crucial role in referring their clients to an independent advocacy scheme, for instance staff employed within the mental health services of Oldham NHS Trust often refer patients to MIND's individual/volunteer advocacy project based within the Royal Oldham Hospital.

Campaigning advocacy

Campaigning advocacy (sometimes called collective advocacy) is where groups and organisations campaign on issues of importance to the people they represent. However, it can only be called advocacy when those directly affected by the issues are directly involved in speaking out for themselves in the campaign or influencing and controlling what others say on their behalf.

Within Oldham, there are many examples, and many of the groups and organisations listed previously also engage in campaigning activity. For instance the Oldham Disability Alliance consult and discuss experiences with groups and take up their issues, reflecting their views, opinions and ideas to those people in a position to change policy.

In practice, the connections between different forms of advocacy are important. For example:

- Citizen advocacy can lead to self-advocacy.
- Self-advocacy groups can play a crucial role in providing the confidence necessary for peer advocacy.
- Staff representation can be vital in linking individual users to a citizen or professional advocate.
- A professional advocate can help in finding a legal advocate if necessary.

Principles and values

There are a number of key principles and values that have been developed within the advocacy movement, which apply to all types of advocacy and all types of user group.

Independence

It is important that there is no conflict of interest between the advocate, whoever they are, whether a paid worker or a volunteer, and the organisation they are advocating to. They must feel and be free to act on the person's behalf. It is equally important that the advocate feels that their first loyalty is to their partner, and not to the organisation providing the advocacy service.

Impartiality

The role of the advocate is to speak on behalf of the person, not on their own behalf, and not to give their own views when they are speaking up on behalf of someone else. This is especially important when there is a conflict, say, between the views of a 'user' and the views of their carer. In this instance it may be necessary for both people to have their own, separate advocates.

Non-judgmental

The advocate is there to help the person say what they want, not to make their own judgement of the advisability of that decision. They need to respect the individual's choice.

Enabling

The process of advocacy is about starting where the person is at and facilitating that person (or group) to articulate their wishes and make decisions on their own behalf. Sometimes this may include helping that person to get information about what is involved, or helping a group of people to listen to each other.

Empowerment

Advocacy is about empowering the person and involves building and giving confidence. This includes providing a reliable, efficient and friendly advocacy service so that the person gets the message that they and their concerns are important to the advocate.

Choice

People should have as much choice as possible about the type of advocacy, which advocate and which service.

Confidentiality

Information that is revealed in an advocacy relationship should not be shared with anyone, unless the person or group wishes it, except in the rare cases where the law requires it to prevent harm to the person or others. This has implications for the keeping of records within an organisation.

Equal opportunities

People should have equal access to advocacy, and should be enabled and supported in this. This means, for example, that an advocacy service should take account of:

● Physical accessibility.
● Language, that is, avoid jargon.
● Cultural sensitivity.

Clarity

The role of an advocate should be made extremely clear to the person and steps taken to see that they understand how advocacy works. Above all, the advocate is on their side and is there for them.

Advocacy in practice

Who can use advocacy?

In principle anyone who needs to speak out for themselves can use advocacy. In practice, advocacy projects and initiatives are usually developed to support particularly vulnerable or disadvantaged groups. In this context, advocacy services are usually set up to support particular users of services. Health authorities and social services departments, for instance, may fund advocacy support for mental health service users, people with learning disabilities, people with physical disabilities and so on. It is important not to be too constrained by these categories as many people will fit into more than one.

Speaking out should be seen as the right of all, not simply of those who need to use services. In order to ensure that people in need, especially the most vulnerable, have access to advocacy, it is important that any advocacy service:

- Advertises itself.
- Provides clear information about what it can offer and the choices available.
- Reaches out to potential users through word of mouth and personal contact, as well as written material.

Who can be an advocate?

Anyone can be an advocate, for themselves or another, providing they follow the principles and values outlined above. The recent *Advocacy: A Code of Practice* developed by the United Kingdom Advocacy Network (NHS Executive 1994) describes the skills of a good advocate in the following way, noting that some of them are innate but that some can be developed through training. They include being able to act as a:

- Recognised independent agent.
- Good interested listener.
- Good communicator.
- Translator into understandable language.
- Support towards independence.
- Reliable and accurate witness.
- Seeker and provider of balanced information.
- Protester for and protector of human rights.

The following list of 'informal advocate roles' is taken from *Citizen Advocacy: A Powerful Partnership* (Butler et al. 1988) but it is a useful list for all forms of advocacy:

- Spokesperson – An advocate who is willing to represent the interests of their partner in situations where his/her rights are at risk of being compromised, neglected or abused.

- Guide – An advocate who assists their partner with practical problem solving. Examples include using public transport, budgeting, acquiring good road sense, shopping, sorting out domestic matters, using the phone.

- Information Aide – An advocate who gives their partner useful information and contacts with the aim of enabling him/her to acquire their entitlements and privileges, for example: general health services, adult education opportunities.

- Financial Advisor – An advocate who gives advice, information and assistance on money issues, for example: welfare benefits, opening a bank account, creating opportunities for their partner to spend his/ her money.

- Monitor – An advocate who is prepared to take on the role of 'watchdog' and monitor their partner's situation, which may be at risk from abuse, neglect and exploitation. This could involve watching out for their partner's health, diet, behaviour and actions of relatives and service workers.

- Neighbour – An advocate who lives in close proximity to their partner and who takes the time to keep an eye on their partner and help out where necessary.

- Enabler – An advocate who, over a period of time, encourages and supports their partner to become more independent and speak up for themselves.

Unless advocates are acting in a legal capacity, where they will have received legal training, it is important that advocates do not take on any legal duties with regard to the person or group they are advocating for. This may change if they have received clear information, and if necessary, training, from the advocacy service about their precise responsibilities; and that both they, and the person they are advocating for, agree to these.

Recruitment and selection of advocates

The criteria for selection of advocates will vary according to the type of advocacy the project is following, and whether it is a paid worker or a volunteer that is being sought. However, there are some key issues which will need to be addressed whatever the process:

- Are you seeking advocate/s who reflect the diversity of people in the local community in terms of age, gender, class, race, etc. or do you want to recruit from a particular group? For example, a project working with Asian people with mental health problems will probably want to recruit from Asian groups.

- Be clear about the principles and values which underpin the work when you are seeking advocates, although you may want to describe and explain these using different words and images than those used in this Code, if that is more appropriate to your client group.

- Be clear about the boundaries of the advocacy relationship, although where you draw them will probably vary according to the type of advocacy, for example, citizen advocacy usually has wider boundaries than, say, legal advocacy.

- Tell potential advocates about the support and training that you offer them – and they will need both support and training. Again, the extent of this will vary according to whether they are a paid worker or a volunteer.

- Consider whether you will ask potential advocates to tell you about any criminal convictions, and whether you will seek a police check. This will help to protect vulnerable people, but there may be reasons why, in some instances, you may not feel such information is appropriate.

Support and training for advocates

Training for advocacy is an essential part of building up an advocacy service, whether this uses paid workers or unpaid volunteers. This section concentrates on the training needs of advocates, whether the advocate is advocating for themselves or another. An important part of the following section is concerned with the training needs of others engaged in the advocacy process.

Advocacy can be a difficult process – it is important to remember that its central aim is to help people speak up for themselves. The advocate will require ongoing support to help them deal with the dilemmas that might arise, while they are happening. For paid workers, this can be provided in a number of ways: regular sessions with their line manager, regular sessions with an outside supervisor or consultant, membership of a support group of advocacy workers, and/or membership of a national advocacy network.

Some of these may be appropriate support mechanisms for a volunteer advocate. In addition volunteers will need regular contact with an advocacy co-ordinator and meetings with their peers.

Training is an essential need as advocates will require knowledge, skills and confidence to help them carry out their roles effectively. Some of these will be innate or already learnt, but others will be new or will need reinforcing. The following is a list of core areas which all advocates will need training in to some degree, regardless of the type of advocacy or their paid/voluntary status:

- Knowledge.

  - definition of advocacy;
  - type of advocacy the project is concerned with (and probably of other types too);
  - acceptance of the principles and values of advocacy;
  - the rights of users within their particular field;
  - responsibilities of advocate and user;
  - structure and organisation of the advocacy service they are involved with;
  - responsibilities of the advocacy project to advocates and users;
  - structures, roles and responsibilities of relevant service agencies, e.g. health services, social services; and
  - relevant contacts.

- Skills.

  - carrying out the role of an advocate;
  - dealing with conflict; and
  - how to use the project and other sources of support and information.

- Attitudes.

  - cultural awareness; and
  - awareness of other differences such as age, gender, disability, sexuality.

In addition, advocates will need training within their particular area, such as the field of learning disability, and their particular type of advocacy, for example, the features of self-advocacy. The training should not have the aim of making them experts in a particular field, but of ensuring that they are clear about their role and know how to handle advocacy situations they may be faced with.

The training may be delivered in a number of ways:

- Informally, in one-to-one situations.
- In-service training courses offered by the project.
- Area-wide training events.
- Participation in outside training courses run by national advocacy networks or outside agencies.

It is important that the training style and methods 'model' the principles and values of advocacy and are clearly structured around developing the knowledge, skills and attitudes listed above.

Setting up an advocacy project

A checklist of steps to take when setting up an advocacy project is described below. These are steps which are important because of the advocacy nature of the project; in addition, the usual procedures that are followed when setting up any community-based project need to be considered. Although the steps are numbered, it is not necessary to follow them in this precise order:

1 Consider precisely who the advocacy service is for – who is the 'client' or user group?

2 Talk with as many potential 'users' as possible right from the beginning about your idea – do they think it is a good one? Are there any concerns and how might these be overcome?

3 Consider who else the project is aimed at – for example, some advocacy projects concentrate as much on work to train and influence service agencies and planners regarding the role of advocacy as they do on providing or supporting direct advocacy for users.

4 Talk with these agencies about your idea to gain their support. Check you would not be duplicating an existing service.

5 Set up a Steering Group to take your idea forward. Make sure this includes members of your 'client group' or users and consider how they can best be supported so that they can participate fully in the group. Try to involve a representative or two from a key service agency who supports the idea.

6 Consider the type of advocacy you want to set up – you do not have to limit yourself to only one type.

7 Consider whether the advocacy scheme needs a paid worker or volunteers or both, and what their roles should be.

8 Consider how support and training will be offered to advocates.

9 Consider a suitable complaints procedure – copies of procedures used by advocacy organisations can be found in *Citizen Advocacy with Older People: A Code of Good Practice* (Dunning 1995) and *A Code of Good Practice for Advocacy in Oldham* (Labyrinth 1996a).

10 Draw up a list of costs you will need to fundraise for and decide how you will seek the funds. Remember to consider worker costs, volunteer

expenses; costs of support and training, practical support costs such as transport, interpreting and so on.

11 Consider who else you need to involve or share your idea with – user groups, other advocacy projects (local and national), other voluntary organisations, representatives from Social Services, the Health Authority, the Health Trust, etc. Think about why you want to involve them, what you want from them and how.

12 Consider where the service should be based. This will depend on the user group and the type of advocacy. Advocacy projects can be based within hospitals, or within independent premises for example. It is important that the base is accessible, friendly and open to users.

13 When you feel you can go ahead with the project, consider the type of management you would like. Make sure it includes user representation and that practical steps are taken to support their full participation.

14 Provide some training right at the beginning for all those involved, from management to volunteers, to explore the principles and values of advocacy. Think through how they can be applied at all levels – with users, with staff, with management and between all these. Try to 'model' advocacy in aspects of the work of the project. Once the project is established, the usual procedures and practices involved in running an effective project will need to be followed.

Case Study: Setting up and running the North Manchester Self-Advocacy Project

North Manchester Self-Advocacy was established in February 1991 to develop and co-ordinate opportunities for people with learning difficulties to speak up for themselves and take more control over their lives. It was financed through a Joint Finance Grant for three years. From the beginning it tried to follow through its philosophy of user involvement at all levels. Before funding was achieved it already had a broad-based steering group which included workers in, and users of, services for people with learning difficulties. The project opened with an office in the local library and the beginnings of a resource library on self-advocacy, a full-time development worker and later on a part-time administrator. In its first year North Manchester Self-Advocacy:

- Provided support to the students' committee at the local adult training centre, and to the users' group at a local day centre.
- Began work with a voluntary organisation providing housing and support for people with learning difficulties and set up users' groups for two of its services, the community service and the residential service.
- Set up and supported a new network group of users of Social Services.
- Recruited and supported volunteer advisers to user/self-advocacy groups.
- Carried out training with users and staff from different services (Social Services, Employment Development, and voluntary organisations).
- Started work to establish a city-wide 'People First', a campaigning self-help and self-run group of people with learning difficulties.
- Carried out consultation on the Community Care Plans with users and the recommendations were submitted to social services.

The following two years saw substantial consolidation of the work in North Manchester, including the establishment and support of more self-advocacy groups and the move to more accessible premises in a community centre. An evaluation of the project after three years analysed why the project had been so successful and what had helped it achieve (Labyrinth 1993a). The project has since been re-funded to cover a wider area. The evaluation identified the following factors as crucial to its success:

- It works at many levels at once with service users, service staff and planners/policy makers. It works at strategic as well as local levels and is combining community development with organisation development. This requires good planning to maintain the balance so that changes are made not only in people's day-to-day lives but in the commissioning, planning and delivery of services. For example, the project supports user groups through independent volunteer advisers, feeds users' views into joint planning processes through a users' co-ordinating group which parallels the Joint Planning Group, and raises awareness and knowledge of users' needs among service providers by providing training sessions.
- Good infrastructure for planning and support through:
  - a high level of individual commitment from all those involved directly with the project;
  - an efficient, organised steering group which involves users in managing the direction of the project, with the support of workers and other group members;

- financial and staff management by the local Council of Voluntary Services which ensures that those tasks are carried out efficiently so that the steering group can get on with managing the work, and that the worker receives good-quality supervision;
- clarity of purpose, aims and objectives from the beginning; and
- initial research and ongoing review of the needs and how to meet them.

● Good ideas for mechanisms for participation which it has put into practice. These include ways of running meetings, providing information and practical back-up and support, e.g. transport and advisers. Each member of the steering group is paired with a member with learning difficulties. The pair go over the minutes after each meeting and over the agenda for the forthcoming meeting to help people feel prepared. Papers for different parts of the agenda are in different colours; drawings and large type are also used.

● Accessible venue which is part of a wider community and leisure centre, on major bus routes and open for long periods.

● Support and co-operation from services (statutory and voluntary) who are open to inviting the project in to help.

● Profile of advocacy has risen recently. In part the project has contributed to this locally but it has also benefited from it.

Monitoring advocacy services

Everybody involved in the advocacy service should be involved in monitoring. This includes:

● Users of the service.
● Advocates.
● Staff.
● Management committee.
● Relevant agencies.

Each project will need to consider how it is going to gather the relevant monitoring information about the service, including the views of these different groups. Some of this information will be about numbers ('quantitative' information), for example the number of people who have used the service, the number of advocates, and so on. It is important that a system is set up right at the beginning so that this sort of information can be gathered easily. Projects will need to consider whose role it is to gather this information, for instance staff, volunteers or management committee members.

Some of this information will be about people's views and opinions of the service ('qualitative' information) and can be gathered in a number of ways:

- Asking people to fill in evaluation forms or questionnaires.
- Talking with groups.
- Talking with advocacy partners separately or together.
- Making a video.
- Discussion at management committee and other meetings.
- Using an outside researcher.

The following is a list of areas that need to be covered in a comprehensive monitoring. Questions within each of these areas can be asked of all groups involved in the service, but should definitely be asked of users and of advocates.

1 Definition – Is the work about helping people 'speak up', or is it more about providing advice or counselling?

2 Types of advocacy – Has the service kept to the type or types of advocacy intended or has it also used other forms of advocacy?

3 Principles and values – For each principle claimed by the project:

- Were they followed in practice? How?
- When were you not sure if they were being followed?
- What support did you receive when you were not sure?

4 Users:

- How did they hear about the advocacy service?
- Were they given any choice in which type of advocacy or which advocate to have?
- What is the composition of users, for example in terms of age, gender, race and so forth?

5 Complaints procedure:

- Did people know about this?
- Did they use it?
- If so, what was their experience?

6 Advocates:

- How did they hear about the advocacy service?
- What is the composition of advocates, for instance in terms of age, gender, race, service user and so on?
- Were they aware of the boundaries of advocacy?
- Did they know about the support and training offered through the project?
- Did they use the support and training offered?
- What was their view of these?

7 Training:

- Did the training cover the areas necessary?
- If not, why?
- What else did it cover?
- Did the training seem effective?

8 Wider support:

- Where did the project receive wider support from?
- What was useful about that support?
- What blocks were there to wider support?
- What else is needed?

9 Benefits – What have been the benefits of advocacy to:

- the user;
- the advocate (they may be the same person);
- the agency;
- the services; and
- the wider community?

Using these questions as a guide, each advocacy service will need to develop their own 'performance indicators' to help them assess their progress.

Strategic approaches to advocacy

Experience throughout the UK suggests that wherever it is practised, the advocacy relationship is, on the whole, an empowering one. It can happen without any support apart from the skills and commitment of an advocate, whether they are advocating for themselves or in partnership with another. However, for advocacy to be accessible to the most vulnerable and to the people most in need, it needs to be supported and resourced. Effective, comprehensive and co-ordinated advocacy helps individuals to speak out. It also helps purchasing organisations fulfil their obligations to involve users in planning and running services.

Strategic support for advocacy requires development of these five elements as described in the diagram below:

- Advocate/user partnership.
- Networking advocacy initiatives.
- Professional alliances.
- Organisation development.
- Central co-ordination and overview.

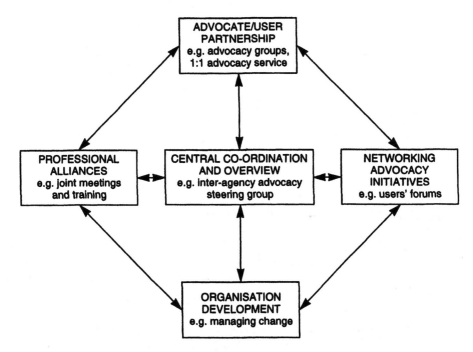

Figure 7.1   Basic elements of a strategic approach to advocacy

Advocate/user partnership

The purpose of supporting this element is to ensure that advocacy is available to those who need it most. Practically, such support can take the form of:

- Funding independent advocacy schemes.

- Encouraging the use of independent local advocacy services and groups by existing service providers.
- Publicising the existence of existing advocacy schemes and groups.
- Funding practical support for advocacy, such as transport costs to get people to advocacy group meetings, publicity costs to advertise the advocacy service to those most in need, and interpretation fees.

Networking between advocacy initiatives

Networking encourages advocacy initiatives to learn from and support each other so that they do not 'reinvent the wheel'. It is also about capacity building, that is, developing the abilities of all those involved in advocacy so that they can sustain that development. Practically this encouragement can take the form of:

- Providing opportunities for paid advocacy workers, unpaid volunteers and users to network with each other, locally and nationally. This includes the provision of training, advocacy newsletters and information sheets, conferences to debate key issues and so on.
- Funding training, good practice materials and other activities designed to build an advocacy infrastructure.
- Setting up and resourcing users' forums and carers' forums with developmental support.

Professional inter-agency alliances

Although it is clear that advocacy needs to be an independent activity, it is also important that professionals and other staff within services, both voluntary and statutory, are given opportunities to build their understanding of the advocacy process and how they can support it, for instance:

- Training staff in the role of an advocate, when advocates are used to help residents in a home which is planned for closure.
- Training staff in the different roles and legitimacy of advocacy and how this connects with their obligations regarding user involvement.
- Joint meetings and training events which explore their roles as service professionals.
- Training can be provided internally, or by advocacy projects, or by an outside agency.

Decision making within organisations

Advocacy has implications for the ways that organisations do things at all levels, not just for the user/advocate partnership. Organisation development will often be needed to help organisations look at their ways of doing things, their decision-making structures and their organisational 'culture'. They may need help to develop ongoing mechanisms for user involvement. This is as important for voluntary organisations as it is for large statutory bodies. This may involve:

- A review of current mechanisms of advocacy and involvement.
- Opening up top-level decision-making meetings to user representation.
- User representatives on management committees.
- Funding/contracting user/carer groups to run and develop their own service.

Central co-ordination and overview

This is important for developing a strategic framework for advocacy. It may involve:

- Establishing a central and multi-agency co-ordinating group to take advocacy forward at all levels within an area.
- Recognition from statutory bodies as well as from voluntary organisations and groups of the importance and function of advocacy.
- Dedicated officer support so that it can play a key information and developmental role regarding advocacy in the area.

Further examples of how advocacy can be supported within a wider service user strategic framework are given in Chapter 14. The model described in that chapter, 'Breadth of support and development needed within a strategic approach to user and carer involvement', lists the development of an advocacy group in a day centre for people with learning difficulties, as an illustration of one method of increasing the participation of users of a specific service. The related Figure 14.3, 'Levels of Involvement and Participation', indicates that advocacy can be used to develop autonomy and empowerment for users.

Taken together, if all five elements of a strategic approach to advocacy are in operation, it will ensure that advocacy is available to those who most need it within a locality or district in a supportive way which promotes good practice. It is interesting and relevant, in this connection, to have a look at the 'advocacy spectrum' developed by Advocacy in Surrey (Clark 1995). This describes a number of activities which can be seen as supporting advocacy. Some of these are relevant to the advocacy partnership, some to organisation development, some to other aspects of the five elements and

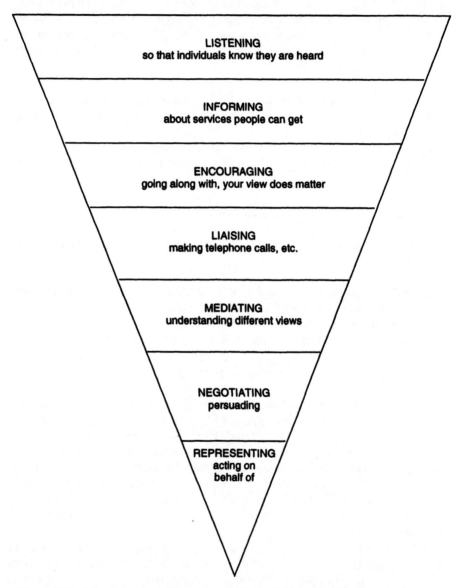

Figure 7.2   The Advocacy Spectrum (adapted from Clark 1995, p. 4)

some to all five. In other words they represent activities relevant to the wider supporters of advocacy (including commissioning and providing organisations, as well as community groups and voluntary organisations).

It may also be useful to look at a model of social services which is user-led and which embodies the principle and practice of advocacy. A fairly recent paper by Jenny Morris (1994) entitled, appropriately, *The Shape of Things to Come?* looks at the growing trend of people who have traditionally been reliant on state services setting up their own organisations and applying for funding to provide what is needed independently. These are organisations controlled either by the people who use them and/or by people who are like those who use them. The following features were deemed to be likely reasons for the existence of such organisations:

- As a result of a process and a wish to bring about radical change.
- As a result of a group of people having a sense of unity and identification and drawing strength from each other.
- Based on a shared commitment to a social model of disability and mental health which determines both the access to, and the nature of, services provided.
- As a response to particular needs at particular times, based on self-identification, flexibility and responsiveness.
- As a way of increasing the choice and control that people have over their lives, involving service users in decisions about how services are delivered and the planning and provision of accountable services.

Discussing user involvement, Morris states that:

> If a statutory or voluntary social services organisation wishes to be user-led, it will:
>
> - Maximise the opportunity for service users to be involved in assessment, care management, service delivery as it affects them as individuals ...
> - Create opportunities for service users to be present at all stages of decision-making which affects groups of service users: that is, planning, purchasing, service delivery, inspection, monitoring and evaluation. [Morris 1994, p. 45]

The report stresses that responsibilities of both statutory and voluntary social services organisations go wider than their existing service users, and into the wider community in taking forward involvement.

A checklist of 'solutions' to the problems experienced by people with learning difficulties when involved in committees and so forth is summarised here from the Autumn 1992 People First's Newsletter. It provides a useful guide for user and carer involvement in general:

- Proper independent support to help with preparation, in meetings and after meetings.
- The supporter is there to support the person, not to take part. The supporter will need to be paid.
- Each person is an individual and will have different sorts of support needs.
- There should be at least two service users on each committee or working group.
- Information needs to be available in a range of formats, e.g. on tape for people who may not be able to read.
- There needs to be a break part way through a meeting, and it should be possible to stop meetings if people need to. Meetings should have a time limit.
- Ground rules such as no jargon, no offensive language, need to be set generally, and at the outset of each meeting.
- People on a committee need to be clear why they want service users on this particular committee; they should be given training by the service users on their needs at the outset, and service users should be given training about what's involved and how to play a real part.

Benefits of advocacy

While it has been argued in this chapter that advocacy is of benefit to all those seeking to empower and involve people in need who use, or potentially could use, services and facilities, it is also of benefit to other key 'stakeholders' in the advocacy process. It is useful to note some of these benefits as they can comprise a powerful argument in pressing for the resourcing and supporting of advocacy. They are listed below.

Benefits to policy makers and funders

- Enables users to be more involved as required in the NHS and Community Care Act (1990) and following government guidelines.
- Ensures services are needs-led.
- Helps to improve quality of life and quality of service as it increases feedback.
- People are more informed about services offered to them.

- Ensures that services are more appropriate and have a higher take-up.

Benefits to service users

- Ensures they have a say.
- Helps them feel involved.
- Helps clear up misunderstandings.
- Helps people get the service they want and need.
- Helps to build confidence.
- Helps to lobby for change.
- Gain respect.
- Access to independent support.

Benefits to service providers

- Problems can be dealt with before they get to complaints procedure levels.
- Extra service to bring in.
- Can support staff views.
- More contented 'users'.
- Help advertise and promote services.
- Value and understanding.
- Help with service development.
- Fit into what government and purchasers want them to do.

Benefits to user advocates and other voluntary advocates

- Skills and self-esteem.
- Employment and career possibilities.
- Gives confidence in own life.
- Empowers self and other users.
- Gives value to own and other people's experience and expertise.
- Reassurance that they would be properly supported.
- Positive role model.
- Link into their motivation to get things changed.

Benefits to carers

- Helps them to support independence and what seems 'best' for their child/relative.
- Helps them to explore their own rights.

- Helps them to find their way round the system, through the spreading of information.
- Helps to ensure that the needs of the user are met.
- Clarifies common areas, where what the carer wants may be the same as what person wants, as well as where it may be different.
- Shows carers they are not on their own in caring for the person.
- Provide information on services.

Note

1 This history is not well documented but this is based on the experiences of a broad range of participants at the first UK conference to bring together different types of advocacy and advocacy groups and workers, 'Speaking Out for Advocacy', held in Bradford in 1995. A report of the event is available from Labyrinth Training & Consultancy, 7–9 Prince Street, Haworth, West Yorks. BD22 8LL; tel.: 01535 647443.

8 Stages in setting up community health projects

Summary

This chapter begins by exploring the main features of community health projects (CHPs). It then moves on to look at the stages that need to be considered when establishing a new project, based on lessons that have been learnt from past projects, through the provision of case studies. Finally a checklist, which can be used both when setting up a new CHP and as part of monitoring progress or trying to address difficulties, is included.

Introduction

Community health initiatives take many forms, but perhaps the most obvious examples of community involvement in health are community health projects. It is difficult to estimate the number of community health projects (CHPs) in the UK as there is no centralised networking or record-keeping. On average there is probably one CHP for each health district (in some there are quite a number, e.g. Newcastle), though some projects may have no formal link with their local health authority. However, what is clear is that the number of projects fluctuates over time, as almost all CHPs are funded through time-limited resources.

Some may be funded through joint finance (e.g. Bradford Community Health Project), some through regeneration money (e.g. Greater Chesterton), a few are funded through health authority contracts directly (e.g. Salford Community Health Project), and some are funded as part of a general contract to a larger organisation, such as a health promotion unit or a community trust (e.g. West Bowling Community Health Action Project in Bradford). Initiatives such as the national lottery and charitable trusts also fund CHPs.

What is a community health project?

When undertaking an audit of community development activity as part of developing a strategy for the health authority, a Bradford working group came up with a diagram to try and distinguish the sorts of projects and initiatives they were particularly interested in (Bradford Health Authority CD Strategy 1995).

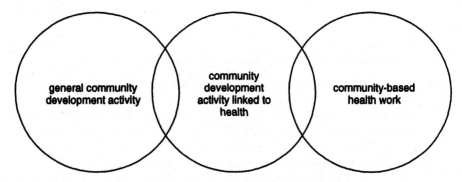

Figure 8.1   Community development and health connections

Initiatives and activity within the circle on the left, that is, general community development activity, obviously overlapped at times with health. For example, a youth development project might include some work in relation to drugs or sporting activities; a housing project might be involved in an anti-dampness campaign that has a health-related aspect. Likewise the activity in the circle on the right, that is, community-based health work, might in some instances lean towards a more community development approach rather than a service delivery model. For example, an initiative such as a stop-smoking group in a local health centre might lead to participants expressing an interest in getting a parent and toddler group going in the neighbourhood. The Bradford group's main concern here was to differentiate between activity or services that happen at community level, but where the power and control stays with health and social care professionals, and those where local people decide for themselves what issues and services they want to develop.

The middle circle, community development activity linked to health, was focused on activity that was both explicitly working to a community development model and was seen by those involved as having a direct relationship to health and well-being. The activities of the two community development and health projects in Bradford (Hutson Street and West Bowling) most easily fitted into this central circle as they clearly fitted both criteria by their very title, but other initiatives were also identified.

Chapter 2 explored the history of community development and health work. A few of the CHPs which were around in those early days in the 1980s when community health initiatives were initially being logged and networked, still remain (for example, Riverside, in Newcastle upon Tyne). They are unfortunately atypical in the fact that they have survived for so many years, albeit changing and adapting to local needs and the changes in the NHS and other services and policies over the years. However, the typical features of a CHP have not changed a great deal over the last 20 years; the same mistakes are being repeated in the way that projects are set up, and the same short-term funding dilemmas still dominate. At a recent meeting of the Steering Group for the Community Health Network (England), about ten workers from local projects were present; of those, around half were coming to the end of their funding, and most were unclear about the future of their employment or the project's work beyond the next three months. Ten years ago a National Community Health Resource Management Committee held three months before the end of a financial year would in all likelihood have illustrated a similar pattern.

The *Guide to Community Health Projects* (CHIRU/LCHR 1987b), described CHPs as using 'a community development approach to their work on health issues. They aim to set up a process by which a community defines its own health needs, considers how those needs can be met and decides collectively on priorities for action' (in Blennerhassett et al. 1989, p. 200).

Typical features of a community health project are:

● Between one and three years of short-term funding.
● Employing between one and three workers, with perhaps an administrative worker as well.
● Workers would usually have a community development background/training, although increasingly workers with community nursing or health promotion training/backgrounds can be seen.
● Based in a particular geographical area, often one which is regarded by local agencies as 'deprived'.
● Possibly working with a particular 'community of interest', for instance women's health projects, black and minority ethnic health projects.
● Working to a WHO-type wide definition of health.

- Working to community development principles and values; for example, the project will usually aim to get local people actively involved in all aspects of the project's work, and in issues that affect the community's health and well-being, as defined by the community.

What does a community health project do ?

Box 8.1   Granton Community Health Project: aims, objectives and activities (Blennerhassett et al. 1989)

Work with small groups
Women and health
Housing and health
Courses for elderly
Family matters
Food and families
Middle years group
Tranquillizers group
Women and food group
Parents and children
Loss and depression

Participatory structures
Pilton elderly forum
Mental health forum
Clinic users group

Audio/visual programmes
'Who knows best?' – The range of advice on feeding babies
'Home Sweet Home' – The effects of dampness on health
'After you leave the surgery' – Psychiatric patients speak out

Training
Sessions with nurses, medical students, community workers, social workers, health visitors etc.

Practical Activities
Fruit and veg. co-op
Keep fit sessions
Relaxation sessions
Counselling
Pensioners' swim club
Pensioner activities
Fitness for big women
Outings

Campaigns
Feet first chiropody campaign
Keep casualty local
Tranquillizers

One-off events
Women's health day
Minor tranquillizers, major problems
Scottish Conference
Elderly Away Day

Granton Stress Centre
A community mental health initiative

A community health project might typically be concerned with identifying local people's health concerns and unmet health needs, and then working with them and local workers and agencies to achieve the changes needed to improve health and well-being in that community. The Granton Community Health Project, which is based in Edinburgh, is one of the atypical projects that has achieved re-funding on a number of occasions and has been able to develop its work and activities successfully for over ten years. One of the project's community development workers set out the range of activities the project was involved with in the late 1980s in an article arguing for more NHS support for CHPs (Blennerhassett et al. 1989, p. 201). The range of activities is not that dissimilar from a CHP in the late 1990s (see previous page).

Making community health initiatives work

Is there a need for a project?

The first question to consider when establishing a CHP is 'Is there a need?' Most projects are set up because local agencies and professionals perceive a need. This may arise because an area or a community of interest show up as having disturbing mortality rates. For example, in one area of Glasgow where a CHP was established, epidemiological data showed that on average people living on that particular outlying estate were likely to die ten years earlier that people living in the next ward just a couple of miles away (Drumchapel CHP 1990). Projects may also feature in areas illustrating other worryingly high levels of deprivation indicators such as levels of unemployment, numbers of single parent households and so forth.

It is very unusual for CHPs to be initiated by local people themselves unless there has already been a history of general community development activity in the area, or with that particular community, and health-related issues have arisen as part of local debates and action. Occasionally, for example through publications, conferences and training events, community activists hear of the activities of CHPs in other parts of the country and start to push for something similar in their locality if they make a connection between other areas with community health projects and concerns in their own neighbourhoods.

However, on the whole most projects are initiated 'top down' because local people are seldom aware of the morbidity and mortality data in relation to their area (and of course in other areas and district/national averages if they are to make comparisons). Even if those statistics do become public knowledge, most people still see health as something that falls within the remit of hospitals, GPs and other health professionals. Decades of an NHS which is oriented towards illness rather than health and well-being have alienated people from their own ability to influence their own health or to take collective action to demand services and support which is focused on keeping people well rather than treating illness. The growth of the public health movement in the UK, for example through the development of the Public Health Alliance, has almost paralleled the growth of the community health movement in this country (although the public health movement has been more successful in maintaining a high national profile and network). Health promotion and public health policies and activities are beginning to influence agendas, from industry and central government down to local people's awareness and consciousness that issues such as poverty, the environment, crime, access to services and resources are all very influential factors on both an individual's and a community's opportunities to maximise their own potential for health and well-being.

CHPs have proved to be very successful in helping to link community agendas and priorities, and those of other local workers and agencies operating in the same geographical area, with health in its widest sense, as well as directly addressing ill-health issues. However, even in communities which are quite well-organised and active, the 'imposition' of a CHP can be most unwelcome, at least initially, and seen as stigmatising the area, as the following case-study illustrates. It is based on a real situation, but for obvious reasons it will remain anonymous and un-referenced.

Case Study: Imposing a community health project

A community health project was put forward by local community nursing managers as part of their input into the process of putting together a bid for City Challenge area status and funding. The area as a whole consisted of three separate neighbourhoods, each of which had very different populations, services and histories of community activity. The City Challenge bid was successful and three CHP workers were appointed, one to each of the three areas. At that point the project base was in a health centre in one of the areas. The worker allocated to area B was based about a mile and a half from the estate she was asked to work on. The estate already had a community centre and a full-time, though very over-stretched, community centre worker. When the CHP worker made contact with the community centre worker and the management committee of the community centre she found that the reception was at best unhelpful and at worst hostile. She floated the idea of moving into the community centre herself, and although this was reluctantly agreed to after some weeks of negotiation, she remained fairly isolated: post went missing, phone messages were never passed on, and so forth. On approaching community nursing staff in the area she found a similar pattern of hostility and also a reluctance to work in partnership.

After some time it became clear that the people involved with the community centre felt that not only this project but other City Challenge initiatives had been foisted on them without any consultation. The welfare rights service offered by the centre was vastly oversubscribed and people would have seen that as a priority. They saw a CHP as a waste of time; health (at least defined in terms of a narrow medical model) was just not a local priority. The community centre building was very overcrowded and the locating of a CHP worker in the building stretched desk and office space beyond what was tolerable. As a new appointment, the CHP worker appeared to be in the luxurious position of just going round the estate and sitting in the community centre chatting, or going off to meetings with her CHP co-workers on the other two estates, whilst the community centre worker was run off her feet.

The community nursing staff had a very different idea about what was needed from what had emerged through their manager's input into the City Challenge bid. There was no base on the estate for any primary care services or support activity and they felt this was desperately needed. They also felt over-stretched and saw a CHP worker as a luxury; what was needed was another community nurse who could ease the workload and deal with the large numbers of already ill and disabled people on the estate.

Unfortunately the CHP worker was not very experienced and was unable to work through the issues outlined above. She took much of the criticism and the unsupportive environment personally, was without any management support, and consequently resigned after three months. The replacement worker was moved to one of the other two areas.

The case study clearly indicates that it is crucial to consult local community groups and local workers from both the statutory and voluntary sectors as part of establishing a CHP. The project may have needed a slightly different remit to complement existing activity in the area, or it may have been accepted as a CHP which could help to address some of the difficulties and concerns of the community centre management committee and worker, and of the community nursing staff, if they had been involved in the setting up of the project, and possibly in the selection of the worker too. The project did not 'fail' because there was not a need for it, but because the remit of the worker and the project was felt to be imposed from outside. There was no negotiation between those holding the statistical data and the management responsibility for the project and the area, and those living and working in the area. Potentially a CHP worker could have offered a lot to the different community groups and service delivery staff in the area (particularly as the project was quite well-resourced) and could have built working alliances around the problems the various paid staff and community activists were facing. However, it would have needed a very skilled and strong worker, with clear and effective line management support, to shift the situation round to a more positive and partnership-oriented working environment after such a disastrous start.

Has the initiative been properly set up?

The case study above gave some indication of poor preparation work before the launch of a community health project. All projects need careful consideration at the preparation stage.

Clear aims and objectives

These might initially be broad and become more specific once the community have had a chance to influence priorities and activity – there are a few examples of projects being established with no aims and objectives, which on the one hand can be seen as giving the CHP workers and the local community an open agenda, but on the other hand can lead to a vague, unfocused project which achieves very little.

A suitable base

Projects also need a suitable base – some projects have their own premises, others share with other voluntary and community groups. The type of premises can influence the activity and networking potential of a new initiative. For example, a very short-term initiative might benefit from sharing premises with an existing community or voluntary project (providing this has been negotiated in advance!) as it may be able to use some of the contacts and credibility of the host project to get its own community health work underway.

Being based in NHS premises such as a health centre can have both advantages and disadvantages. Some projects, such as the Wells Park Health Project have worked in close partnership with local GPs, nurses and other primary care staff with whom they share premises, without having to compromise the community development approach to their work. The health centre is a positive and open building and it is easy for people to drop in to the CHP. In other instances projects have been based in the far reaches of health centre buildings, with no working relationship with the primary care staff based in the building and no direct access for local people (who have to negotiate with the centre receptionists to get through to the project offices!). In these cases, having an NHS base is at best irrelevant and at worst off-putting for local people.

Some projects have gone for shop front-type premises, and this has worked well as a means of drawing people in, both because of the window displays, and because such premises are often in areas with other shops and facilities frequented by local people. Such buildings can, however, be a staffing and security nightmare. If the project only has one or two staff, the drop-in nature of the building can lead to becoming very focused on the base rather than undertaking outreach work and linking into other community buildings.

There seem to be increasing numbers of projects which are based some distance from the geographical area they are set up to serve. This is partly as a result of projects serving several areas and thus not having a base in every one, but it is also about the growth of statutorily funded CHPs who then inevitably end up based in the offices of their organisation. If the organisation is serving a whole town or district then it is unlikely that the central offices will be based in the areas where CHPs are felt to be needed. There can be some advantages to this, for example being based closer to the centres of power and decision making, and a central base can offer ways of networking with other workers and accessing information and contacts that more isolated projects may be excluded from. However, not being based in the area one is supposedly working within means relying on there being other premises that can be accessed for group work, crèches, etc., which can also have cost implications. It can also mean that the project has very little presence or visibility and certainly usually excludes local people from dropping in or getting involved as volunteers with the day-to-day running of the project.

Appropriate staff and structure

The appointment of appropriately qualified/experienced staff and clear team roles and accountability structures is crucial – there are growing numbers of CHPs staffed by people from community nursing backgrounds with little or no experience of community development work. This can lead to problems for their own professional competence and confidence, and can lead to tensions in teams which are a mixture of health professionals and community development workers. This is not to say that some people from health professional backgrounds do not make excellent CHP workers, nor that if offered training and support most will not be able to make the shift in roles from service delivery and 'expert' to encouraging the community to identify its own priorities and concerns and for people to trust to their own experience as well as professional expertise.

Multi-disciplinary teams can be difficult, particularly if line management and accountability structures are messy or not addressed (for example, community nurses may be supervised under the nurse management structures even if they are working within CHPs; salary scales and even holiday entitlement may be different between staff with the same job descriptions if some are qualified nurses and others are qualified community development workers). The personnel systems and structures within NHS trusts in particular can lead to problems with treating staff from different professional backgrounds as part of the same team for management purposes. This quote from an evaluation report for a CHP in the English Midlands illustrates how the difficulties above can manifest themselves:

> The manner in which the project workers were recruited contributed to their failure to work as a group. Each of the four was recruited in a different way. Only the co-ordinator was recruited through advertisement, short listing and interview. The part-time community nutrionist [sic] had already taken up post by internal appointment before the co-ordinator was appointed. The part-time health visitor was appointed without the co-ordinator being involved in the decision. However, the part-time secretary was appointed by interview with the co-ordinator involved in the selection. Subsequent conflicts of personality and aims, which often arise in CDH projects, were particularly difficult to deal with because of lack of cohesion among the workers from the start ...
>
> Day-to-day management of the project had been intended to be the responsibility of the co-ordinator but, because of the ambiguity of his role amplified by the methods of recruitment, in fact the workers tended to work independently with little co-ordination.
>
> The strategy board adopted a very loose style of overall supervision of the project. This was partly deliberate in order to allow the workers latitude to adapt their work to the needs and opportunities they found, and because the Strategy Board felt that there were no well founded principles so the project had to be experimental. When disputes did arise they were mainly dealt with informally by Strategy Board members in one-to-one conversations with individual workers. [Luck and Jesson 1995, pp. 25–26]

A key lesson from this project is that community development is not something that anyone can do without previous experience and training, and also that team working is crucial.

Funding and budgets

Projects need to cover staffing and accommodation costs but also to have extra finance available for development work with groups and local people (to hire meeting rooms, pay for crèches, get publicity materials printed, and so forth). An amount for staff training should also be included. CHP workers can be very isolated and the opportunity for informal learning, for example, by visiting other projects around the country and attending relevant conferences and training events, can both boost staff morale and bring in ideas and resources. Local people may also want to access training and networking events and opportunities as they get more involved in community health work and groups.

Even when funding is adequate there is a need for a clear budget breakdown which is accessible to everyone involved with the project. One CHP operated for the first six months without any budget breakdown – the line manager had left just as the project workers were appointed. This had major effects as they were unable to ascertain how much money remained after their salaries were paid, nor were they able therefore to purchase basic requisites such as desks and phones, let alone have stationery printed or pay for crèches and meeting room hire.

A final cautionary note, drawn from the experience of many small projects, is that most statutory organisations (and the lottery too) often pay over funding at least three months in arrears. This puts projects in impossible situations with regard to money management. The accounts departments of statutory agencies are also often not geared up for making small payments, either in advance or quickly afterwards, and claiming can often be very bureaucratic and involve endless form-filling. This can be very problematic when, for example, trying to pay crèche workers or meet people's travel costs. Having a development fund that the workers can manage and allocate themselves, albeit with proper record-keeping and accountability, can make the difference between keeping and losing local volunteers and group members. Projects based in the voluntary sector seldom have the same problems accessing these small, but crucial, pots of money as those based directly within statutory organisations.

Does the project have sufficient status to effect change?

Some projects have very clear aims and objectives, but are then set up in such a way that it is difficult to meet those aims and objectives, either because the funding period or the resources are insufficient, or because the status of the workers and the project are not sufficiently senior, nor located within decision-making structures which can effect change. The case study below illustrates this. Again, it is based on another real-life situation but is presented anonymously.

Case Study: How not to set up a community health project

The project was set up as part of a City Challenge initiative (a different one to the earlier case study). This is not to imply that regeneration-type initiatives necessarily lead to the setting up of poorly planned projects. They have been the source of a lot of newly developed CHPs over the last five years and some crucial lessons have now hopefully been learnt. The increased emphasis in SRB regeneration bidding on a great deal of community involvement and inter-sectoral partnership input into bids makes it more likely that project planning will be properly thought through.

The CHP was set up with one three-quarter-time and one full-time worker, located within a Community Health Council building, a few miles from the area to be focused on (this itself presented other problems of the type explored above in the section on premises). A small voluntary management committee was established which included someone from the CHC and some local voluntary organisations, plus a few local workers from other agencies in the area served by the project.

One of the main aims of the project was to allow people from the local area to feed into the planning and purchasing decision making of the health authority and of social services (in relation to community care). However, no one from either of these organisations was involved with the project management, and thus there were no formal relationships between the project, the health authority and social services. When representatives were sought the people who came along were of insufficiently high status to effect any real influence on their organisation's planning or priorities.

No one from City Challenge (the funders) attended the management committee either, consequently all monitoring and liaison was done outside of the management committee structures. This became particularly problematic for the CHP workers when the expectations of the City Challenge initiative (and ultimately the Department of the Environment) were found to be somewhat different to the priorities and monitoring sought by the management committee, which in turn did not really fit with local people's priorities.

This situation was eventually resolved to a large degree, but it took over a year and the involvement of external consultants to remedy the structural, power and status issues.

Linking the project with the aims and priorities of key agencies

Given the pace of change in the statutory services over the last few years it is not surprising that personnel changes in organisations such as local authorities and health authorities can be very extensive. It is therefore important that local CHPs, if they are reliant on statutory funding or if they need to find channels and mechanisms to enable local people to influence services and policies, can link themselves to organisations by way of policies and not just key individuals. One project in Bradford has tried to do just that, by using an evaluation to explore the ways in which the project links to health and local authority priorities. This was partly stimulated by having six changes in the liaison contacts within the statutory organisations over an 18-month period. It was clear that the project needed to link to policies and areas of priority development, not just to individuals, as these relationships could not be relied on. The section of the report which looks at the links is reproduced below as it is likely to be relevant to CHPs and statutory organisations in other parts of the country too.

Policy and strategic implications

It is evident that the work of the project has direct links to Bradford Health Authority, Trust and Social Service policies and priorities including primary based care; health promotion; community involvement and consultation; work with children and young people; black and minority ethnic communities; devolution of nursing management to community nursing teams; neighbourhood forums; area based commissioning involving GPs. Furthermore the project has plans to expand and develop many of these areas ...

The future

The professional workers and project users have clearly identified the activities that the project now needs to undertake. These are:-

- develop and increase the links with GPs;
- develop and increase the links with community nursing staff;
- continue to link into multi-agency initiatives in the Bradford 5 area;
- continue to link the community into initiatives such as the 'One-Stop' shop and Neighbourhood Forum;
- forge stronger links with local GP commissioning group(s);
- forge stronger links with Bradford Health Authority planners and purchasers;

- seek funding for a black/Asian worker;
- seek funding for increased welfare rights support work;
- continue to support groups and activities identified by local people;
- continue development work to support initiatives such as Credit Union, Play schemes and so on that can help with issues around poverty and health;
- expand work in relation to young people and health in partnership with the new Youth Action Project;
- develop, with Bradford Health Authority an evaluation protocol for community development health work across Bradford; and
- once the Horton Park Centre is functioning there will be a need to review the project's direct involvement. [Kilminster 1996, p. 16]

A community health project checklist

The remainder of this chapter is organised as a 'checklist' to use either when setting up a community health project, when dealing with problems or difficulties in performance, or when reviewing or evaluating a project. It is intended as a way of highlighting issues that need addressing, ideally at the outset of a CHP, but may also help to focus on why certain problems are emerging, or goals are not being reached once a project is up and running. The checklist is organised around a series of questions, and contains both further questions to aid the next stages of development and some suggestions for action.

Table 8.1   Community Health Project checklist

ASSESSING THE NEED	ACTION?	
	Yes	No
Has the idea to explore setting up a CHP come from a single agency?	If yes, might there be other agencies and groups who would want to work in partnership on this initiative – how might you get them involved?	If no, have arrangements been made to establish a multi-agency 'steering group'; have issues in relation to roles, relationships and expectations been explored?

Table 8.1 continued

ASSESSING THE NEED	ACTION?	
	Yes	No
Has the idea come from local people or out of existing local community development work?	If yes, how can local people hold on to the initiative; can the project be set up and run with a local voluntary management committee; should local people also seek the involvement of local professionals and agencies?	If no, how can local people be involved in the next stages (audit and needs assessment) to get their views and ideas?
Has an audit of what's already available in the local area been undertaken? Has there been a needs assessment of what a community health project would add to the area, and to local people?	If yes, does this indicate that a CHP would complement other activity in the area?	If no, who might be in a position to undertake this and feed back the findings?
Are there clear aims and objectives for the project (i.e. what it will achieve, and how)?	If yes, are they based on the audit and needs assessment, or do they need to be refined to take into account the finds of that work?	If no, can broad aims and objectives be set from the audit and needs assessment exercises; who needs to be involved in setting them?

Table 8.1 continued

GETTING THE PROJECT STARTED	ACTION?	
	Yes	No
Is there an existing suitable base for a project?	If yes, when will it be available and for how long?	If no, is there an opportunity to convert premises or purpose build (e.g. a portacabin?)
Has there been an assessment of the resources that will be needed to meet the aims and objectives (e.g. numbers and roles of staff; type of base needed, etc.)	If yes, is it likely that sufficient resources will be available? If not it may be necessary to refine and narrow down the aims and objectives.	If no, who might be in a position to undertake this?
Is there money for a training/staff development fund in the budget?	If yes, how will this be allocated; who will determine training needs and opportunities?	If no, is it too late to include this? How else might staff access training and development (e.g. via free places on training run by other local organisations; by applying for grants and bursaries)?
Has there been an assessment of how much funding is needed?	If yes, does this meet the total need for resources as determined above?	If no, who might be in a position to cost out the various resources identified above?

Table 8.1 continued

GETTING THE PROJECT STARTED	ACTION?	
	Yes	No
Has there been an assessment of possible funders and pros and cons of different types of funding?	If yes, are there any limits or conditions attached to certain types of funding that contradict the aims and objectives of the project? Are you willing to compromise? Is the project to be funded by a single or multiple sources? If multiple how will the relationships with and between different funders be managed?	If no, who is in a position to do this and feed back the results? It is important to think this through before accepting funding from sources or combinations of sources that may lead to problems in the future.

SECURITY OF FUNDING	ACTION?	
	Yes	No
Is the length of funding likely to be adequate to meet the project's aims and objectives?	If yes, keep under review.	If no, either revise aims and objectives or see next question below.
If funding is short-term, is there a plan for applying for re-funding?	If yes, see next question below.	If no, consider putting a plan together soon after the beginning of the project as statutory funders often budget at least nine months to a year ahead; lottery/ charitable trust bids often need quite a long run in, too.

Table 8.1 continued

SECURITY OF FUNDING	ACTION? Yes	No
Has someone taken on/been given the responsibility for co-ordinating the re-funding strategy?	If yes, do they have the time, contacts and skills to undertake this task?	If no, then either the task will fall to the workers to seek re-funding (see below) or it may get left until a crisis looms in which case deadlines (see above) may have been missed.
If the worker(s) are to take responsibility for re-funding, has this been taken into account in terms of the rest of their work and responsibilities?	If yes, keep this under review; workers on short-term contracts can spend a lot of time on fundraising to the detriment of their main tasks and roles. Fundraising is really a management role.	If no, then the project manager or management committee will need to take the lead responsibility, bearing in mind the issues above.
Is there a clear relationship between the evaluation process and possible re-funding; i.e. are you finding out what existing and potential funders may want to know?	If yes, this will mean you have a very clear agreement between the project and its funders and hold regular feedback/review sessions. Are the people sufficiently senior to know about and be able to influence funding policy and decision making?	If no, there is a danger that all the project's record-keeping, monitoring and evaluation may be in vain if existing and potential funders are working to different criteria in terms of priority setting and funding.

Table 8.1 continued

SUPPORT and MONITORING	ACTION?	
	Yes	No
Have arrangements been made for keeping records?	If yes, is everyone involved clear about who is keeping records, what sort of records, and why?	If no, agreement needs to be reached as per the 'yes' column.
Has an evaluation model been agreed on?	If yes, are additional resources needed for the evaluation and where might they be forthcoming from?	If no, the project needs to determine how it is going to be evaluated; by whom; at what stage in its development; what the time and cost implications are; the purpose of the evaluation (see Chapter 10 on evaluation).
Are there mechanisms in place for feeding back to/regularly reviewing progress with funders?	If yes, are the people at the right levels in their respective organisations to influence decision making in relation to the project's future?	If no, mechanisms need to be put in place, ideally involving periodic face-to-face meetings as well as written reports.
Is there clarity about workers' and management roles and responsibilities?	If yes, this needs to be kept under regular review and any overlaps, gaps or confusion sorted out as soon as it comes to light.	If no, time needs to be devoted to getting this clear, perhaps with the help of an external facilitator, otherwise problems will inevitably arise.

Table 8.1   continued

PROJECT STATUS	ACTION?	
	Yes	No
Is there clarity about roles and responsibilities of different team members?	If yes, is this verbal or written down (staff may change); is there a hierarchy or is the team of equal status? How will decisions be made and work allocated?	If no, this needs to be sorted out at an early stage, particularly in project teams with all staff of equal status, and/or multi-disciplinary teams who may come into the project with different skills, approaches and attitudes to community health work.
Has a relationship been established between the project and the agencies and individuals it may need to influence?	If yes, then it is likely that either the project is already well-developed, or that there has been a lot of clear thinking when the project has been established.	If no, then the aims and objectives need to be revisited; which agencies and individuals will be key to the successful meeting of these aims (e.g. Stakeholder Analysis, see Chapter 11). Getting mechanisms in place can take a great deal of time but may pay off in the end.

Table 8.1 continued

PROJECT STATUS	ACTION? Yes	No
Have key agencies made links between their aims and objectives and those of the project?	If yes, then the project is likely to have been very successful (!!) or have been initiated by that agency (or agencies) in order to help meet its own aims and objectives.	If no, the key agencies may need some help with making the links; it can be useful to get hold of documents such as the Community Care Plan (social services); Purchasing Plan (health authority) any community development or public consultation policy documents etc. and produce a short paper showing how the project can feed into key agency policies and priorities (see Kilminster 1996)
Do the agencies have clear structures and systems to enable the project to feed in needs and ideas emerging from the work?	If yes, either the agencies will have developed their community/public involvement policies and structures to a very sophisticated degree, or there will be one or two very useful individual contacts who have been able to have the vision and clout to 'oil the wheels'.	If no, start by trying to identify sympathetic and influential individuals and also by building up support from other voluntary and community projects to put pressure on agencies to develop mechanisms to allow for 'bottom-up' needs and ideas to be fed into service planning and policy and priority setting (see Chapter 14).

9 Participatory health needs assessment

Summary

This chapter looks at the reasons for the growth of interest in participatory needs assessment, and explores the different ways that communities can be involved in identifying needs and in working in partnership with key local agencies to find ways of meeting those needs. Ways of determining which areas to focus on for a needs assessment exercise are discussed, and case studies of both the process of undertaking a participatory needs assessment, and in selecting a geographical area are included.

Introduction

When the 1990 legislation to separate out health purchasing from health service providers came onto the statute book, it brought with it the concept of the health authority as the 'champion of the people'. Implicit in this idea was the notion that health authorities must assess the needs of their local populations, in order to prioritise their spending against local health needs.

Traditionally most information about health need has been assumed from epidemiological and census data, which is collected by health authorities and other agencies at district levels, and nationally by the Department of Health and other government departments and agencies. Priorities for health authority spending are still largely set centrally, but increasingly authorities are beginning to look at ways of assessing need, not just based on statistical data, but also from the perspectives of local people. This is called 'participatory health needs assessment'.

151

As has been discussed in previous chapters, the 1992 NHS Management Executive publication of *Local Voices* was influential in providing both a policy document and a practical guide for health authorities. It also highlighted that the scale of change that was envisaged if local people were going to be effective partners in determining local health policy and priorities required 'a radically different approach' (p. 1).

Further policy changes and developments have seen the merging of Family Health Service Authorities (FHSAs) and health authorities and now the development of Primary Care Groups (PCGs) taking forward a 'primary care-led NHS' (though in reality the acute care sector is still very dominant). In practice it means that the formal role of health authorities has been widened. They are responsible not just for the purchasing of health care but for the overall health and well-being of their local population through coordination of Health Improvement Programmes. There have also been other policy developments which have led to practical change implications over the last few years, such as the development of the notion of community care (for example, 'Care in the Community', the NHS and Community Care Act 1990); more emphasis on health promotion (*Our Healthier Nation*, Department of Health 1998); a much stronger focus on the need for the NHS to work in partnership with other agencies (the concept of 'Healthy Alliances'); the increased importance of primary care ('PCGs'), and local people's involvement in needs assessment, planning, prioritising, and decision making (for example, *Local Voices*).

The NHS Executive have promoted the idea that the prime aim of effective purchasing is to improve the health of local people (not simply to purchase health care services). History has shown us that most improvements in health, quality of life and mortality and morbidity data have come about by much wider changes than simply treatments for illness and disease, for example, improvements in sanitation, housing and other such social and environmental factors. Thus, in order to carry out their purchasing and commissioning functions effectively, health authorities/commissions need to develop 'healthy alliance' partnerships with other agencies and to actively involve local people.

Participatory needs assessment in context

There are five main perspectives which influence health authorities' policy priorities and spending plans. These are illustrated in Figure 9.1 below.

This chapter is mainly concerned with exploring ways of identifying, and ensuring action from, local people's perspectives.

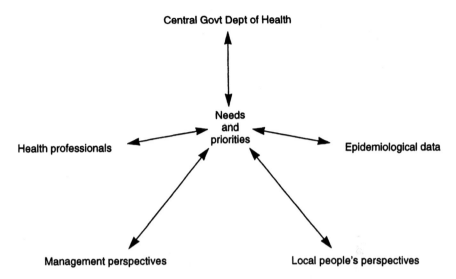

Figure 9.1   Perspectives influencing health authorities' priorities and spending plans

In the early days of the purchaser/provider split, many health authorities set out with positive intentions to reach out to local people, to draw in their views and opinions, and collect feedback. However, the processes used were not, on the whole, very participatory.

For example, one health authority in East Anglia sent out questionnaires to almost one-fiftieth of its local population, asking for people's satisfaction ratings on around eight services. Each respondent was asked to score the services on five grades between poor to very satisfactory. They obtained a reasonable response rate, but in retrospect felt they had only scratched the surface in terms of beginning to engage with local people. They found out that most people considered the services to be satisfactory or very satisfactory, but had no notion of whether people were grading from personal experience or not, nor whether there were any specific areas of service provision, within an overall service, which needed improvement. Surveys such as this can give some crude general indication of satisfaction with what already exists, but not about unmet need or wider perspectives. They also had no means of having an ongoing dialogue with local people, nor of identifying people's priorities.

In some areas of work, mental health for example, epidemiological sources may give little indication of the needs or experiences of local people. A report for Stoke-on-Trent City Council by Colin Thunhurst and Sjoerd Postma (1989), noted:

Where further development of additional data sources is undoubtedly required is in relation to subjective or 'soft' health data. We currently know next to nothing about the community's own perception of its health. Subjective perceptions can be invaluable, not only as early indicators of health problems that may emerge in a 'harder' form later, but also as an *essential* pre-condition for meaningful community development planning.

Subjective data can also be invaluable in filling another data gap that is highlighted by our study. That is in relation to mental health. Mortality data, and even that little morbidity data that exists, relates almost exclusively to physical ill-health. As such, psychological well-being, arguably even more important in evaluating the life experience, remains lacking. [pp. 32–33]

In an internal document, North Staffordshire Health Authority note that both the concepts of 'health' and 'need' are ill-defined, which means that there is no well-developed and coherent model of 'health needs assessment'. The process should:

... encompass all aspects of health and not just focus on assessment of need for health care services. This means that the methodology has to be more than the traditional 'epidemiological' approach ... but should also look at issues of social and mental well-being, physical fitness, and self esteem for example and at whether social and environmental conditions are conducive to health.[1]

Over the last three to four years participatory methods have been developed, and are being taken forward by a number of organisations, which are grounded in qualitative research and community development methodology. A number of examples of such approaches will be referred to in the rest of the chapter.

Getting participation at all stages in the needs assessment process

The following checklist can be used to help explore how local people's involvement can be obtained at all stages in a needs assessment process. This is particularly important when taking forward needs assessment in ways that are rooted in community development approaches, with local people's participation being central throughout the process.

Needs assessments vary in the methodology used. Sometimes focus groups are the main way of interacting with local people; in some instances questionnaires or semi-structured interviews are used. There are numerous examples of health authorities employing people such as market researchers or other social science-based agencies and consultants to undertake research in local geographical communities, or with communities of interest. However, although such approaches elicit information from local people, they seldom engage local people's participation; people remain passive respondents, rather than active participants.

Figure 9.2 below sets out the different stages at which a participatory approach to needs assessment should, and can, engage the commitment and involvement of local people. Ideally, at each stage the levels of participation should be at or towards the 'high' end of the continuum.

The checklist can be used as a planning tool, to help you think through how to achieve participation at each stage of the process, and also as a review tool, to check back what has actually been accomplished.

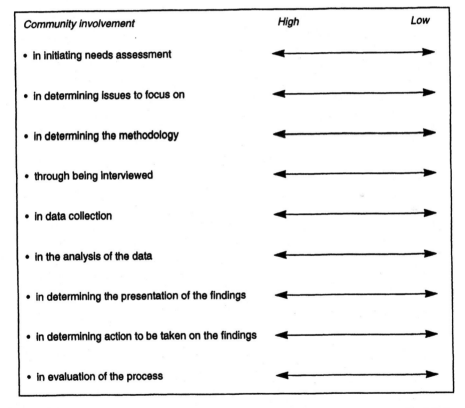

Figure 9.2   Local participation in the needs assessment process: a checklist

The case study that follows is an example of how local people were able to play an active part in the process of a needs assessment in their local area.

Case Study: Involving local people in a needs assessment (Oldham)

In Oldham, the Health Authority had established a 'Local Voices' Steering Group, to co-ordinate work around eliciting information from, and the involvement of, local people in health. The Steering Group was comprised of representatives of different departments within the Health Authority, plus people from the Local Authority, NHS Trusts and Community Health Council.

This multi-agency group decided that an initial piece of work should be undertaken to help the group get focused on its task. A participatory needs assessment on the Limeside estate was chosen. This was partly because the community trust already had a community development and health project in the area; partly because the area was known to have relatively poor health and high levels of deprivation in comparison with the district as a whole, and partly because the estate was felt to have clear geographical boundaries and to be a definable 'community'.

Outside consultants (Labyrinth) were appointed after a tendering process. An initial workshop was organised for the local community, to inform people about the proposed needs assessment, and to ask for their ideas, experiences and, hopefully, their involvement. Invitations were delivered door-to-door and via community groups and venues. Lunch and child care were provided, and the timings for workshops were organised around school hours. This first workshop introduced local people to the idea of needs assessment by showing a section of a video made by residents from an estate in Glasgow (Drumchapel Community Health Project 1990) who had undertaken their own needs assessment. This was followed by small group discussions, for Limeside residents to share their perceptions about what affects health locally, and what sort of action could help to improve local people's health and well-being. This gave us the basis of the outline for what issues to look at in the needs assessment.

Altogether 28 people came to the first workshop; of these 23 were local residents and five were local workers (school nurse, health visitor, and so on). At the end of the session people agreed to meet again a couple of weeks later to look at what sort of needs assessment methods to use. People also agreed to tell neighbours, family and friends about the next meeting.

The turn-out for the next meeting was down to 22, but included several new people. After much discussion about the pros and cons of different methods, the group agreed that if they wanted to get a good cross-section of the people living in Limeside they would need both to undertake group discussions with people involved in the range of community groups on the estate, and also do some door-to-door interviewing. In addition it was decided to bring the health bus onto the estate for three days to be used as a drop-in for anyone who wanted to call in and fill in a questionnaire.

Based on this discussion the consultants went away and drafted a questionnaire that could be used for the door-to-door interviews and an interview schedule, with some outline headings, to use in group discussions.

A training workshop followed for everyone who wanted to carry on with the work, and actually become interviewers. Altogether, 14 local people and eight local workers undertook interviewing with individuals and/or groups. The training included looking at safety, confidentiality, and practical issues such as where to collect and drop off the questionnaires. The participants also had a chance to try out the questions and to practice interviewing people. They gave lots of practical feedback about particular questions which were felt to be unclear, or that they would not feel comfortable with.

A mail drop was undertaken across the whole of the estate, advising people that someone might be calling round with a questionnaire, and telling them where the health bus would be. All the interviewers wore security badges and most worked in pairs, especially for the group interviews.

A three-and-a-half-week period was set aside to undertake the interviews. The interviewers all met together part-way through the process to share how things were going. Once all the questionnaires were in, the consultants undertook some initial analysis, and wrote a draft report. This was presented back to the local interviewers, and any other local people who wanted to be involved, in order to determine priorities for action, and to decide on the best ways of feeding back to the estate as a whole. A final report was then drafted, and an exhibition display plus a news-sheet summarising the findings were put together. The news-sheet was delivered to all households on the estate.

Finally the report was presented to a multi-agency forum of decision makers to get their support for, and commitment to, taking action on some of the needs and priorities identified (Labyrinth 1993d).

Who should a needs assessment have as its focus?

Research undertaken by the authors of this book for the NHS Executive a couple of years after the *Local Voices* document was launched (Labyrinth 1993b) indicated that there were four main ways in which organisations, and in particular health authorities, were approaching the concept of 'local people'.

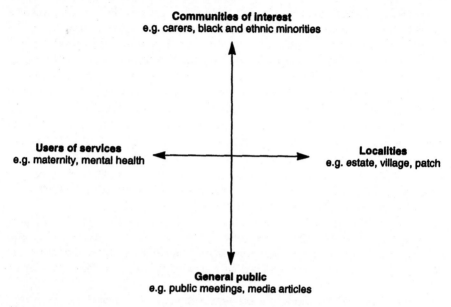

Figure 9.3   Four approaches to categorising local people

There are a number of reasons to consider targeting particular groups of people when undertaking a needs assessment: These include:

- Only recent service users or people who live in a specific area are likely to have a useful view about it.
- People are much more likely to respond if they feel it is relevant to them.
- Narrower focus means more time can be put into preparation, publicity and development.
- It is easier to analyse the findings if some of the variables can be controlled.
- It is easier to make changes if initial boundaries are fairly tight and well drawn.[2]

When selecting a geographical area for undertaking needs assessment, a number of factors need to be considered. Quite commonly areas are selected because local statistics such as morbidity and mortality data and census materials indicate higher than average levels of deprivation, and poorer health and earlier average age of death. The case study below looks at this approach in relation to one area within North Staffordshire.

Case Study: Focusing on areas of high deprivation and poor health (North Staffordshire)

North Staffordshire Health Authority is part of the NHS and as such is part of all the national changes and developments explored in earlier chapters. There is also a commitment to look at ways to tackle inequalities in health. The Authority has developed a plan of work to take forward what it calls 'A Multi-City Action Plan on Urban Primary Health Care Systems'. The plan focuses on six particular electoral wards which, statistics indicate, have populations that on average experience poorer health and higher deprivation than other parts of North Staffordshire. These have been designated 'Health Action Areas'.

Three 'Healthy Alliance' workers have been appointed by the Health Authority, based in the Health Promotion Department, who link to 'Healthy Alliance' partnerships formed with the three local authorities that cover North Staffordshire. The partnerships bring together local authority, private and voluntary sector representatives to look at common ways forward for preventing ill health and promoting better health. Tunstall, which is a small township within Stoke-on-Trent, comes within the remit of the Stoke-on-Trent Healthy Alliance Partnership.

'Health Profiles' had been compiled for each of the other five Health Action Areas, bringing together statistical data, details of existing services, and the views of some local workers about what is needed in terms of additional resources to improve health and well-being in the area. However, less was known about Tunstall than the other five areas and it was felt pertinent to undertake more in-depth work in Tunstall, including contacting and involving local workers and local residents.

In July 1989 a report was produced for Stoke-on-Trent City Council entitled *Health Profile of the City of Stoke-on-Trent* (Thunhurst and Postma 1989). The researchers noted that people's health in Stoke-on-Trent was, as a whole, considerably worse than the overall national position, with mortality (death) rates 25–30 per cent above comparable national rates. Data relating to Tunstall needed to be understood within this context. However, it is true to say that Tunstall came out as having some fairly poor morbidity and mortality statistics, even given the overall poor position of Stoke-on-Trent as a whole.

The 'Health Profile' report explored the relationship of mortality to social and economic deprivation. The authors noted that the precise nature of the relationship between poverty and ill health is not universally agreed, but concluded that, 'Whatever the exact links in that relationship, they are clearly present in the City of Stoke-on-Trent today.'

As well as reaching that conclusion for the City as a whole, the 'Health Profile' report also noted that at ward and neighbourhood levels, 'there is a very clear relationship between those areas suffering the poorest health experience and those areas suffering from measurable material deprivation' (p. 26). The data available for Tunstall showed both higher than average deprivation statistics and higher than average mortality figures.

The report's authors acknowledged that much lies outside the control of the respective authorities in terms of elimination of social and economic deprivation and its consequences for ill health, and that pressure needs to be brought on national and international bodies. However, they also note that:

> ... there are a number of actions that the authorities can take now to ensure that current services, and potential services, delivered by each acknowledge and respond to the existence of poverty and social and economic deprivation as a cause of the current levels of ill-health experienced within the City. [p. ii]

The 'Health Profile' report contained a number of recommendations. These focused specifically around what they termed 'an inter-agency community development approach'. Six years later, an inter-agency community development approach was explored in Tunstall, beginning initially with a participatory needs assessment which was undertaken in 1995 (Labyrinth 1996e) and the multi-agency 'Tunstall Health Forum' formed out of the needs assessment work, which is following up the findings and recommendations.

Thus, indications that the area may be suffering poorer health and higher levels of deprivation than most neighbouring areas is one factor often taken into consideration when considering where to focus a participatory needs assessment. Other factors, explored in the remainder of this chapter, to take into account are:

- Time limits on the needs assessment process.
- Existence of community groups and networks.
- Existence of any cross-agency forums and networks.
- Past history of research/needs assessment in the area.
- Priority given to the area by other agencies.
- Definition of a 'community'.

Time limits

If time is short then the methodology used and the area to be focused on will have to be carefully selected. If there has been very little history of community development in the area, then it may initially be difficult to contact and get local people involved in the needs assessment process. We feel that at least nine months to a year is needed to undertake initial outreach work, contacting people and building up trust as well as then moving on to get involvement in the needs assessment itself. Methods such as 'rapid appraisal' may need to be used rather than a more in-depth participative survey such as that used in the Oldham case study.

Existence of community groups and networks

It is always much easier to undertake a needs assessment if a range of community groups and networks already exist. Such groups give ready-made initial access points to particular sectors of the community (for example, parents via a mother and toddler group, older people via a pensioners' group, a cross-section of people via a tenants' organisation, young people via a youth centre, and so on). Community groups can be both a direct source of involvement (for example, they can become 'focus groups') or can be a way of getting together a cross-section of the community to be involved in a needs assessment (if each group sends along representatives to a planning group, for example). People involved in community groups also usually have other friends, family and neighbours who can be encouraged to get involved.

If an area has very few community groups and networks in existence, inevitably a needs assessment process will take longer as it will be harder to contact and involve local people. There may need to be a development role in helping to get groups started as well as getting participation in the needs assessment. Areas with little community infrastructure may be the ones that most need a participatory needs assessment, which can in itself be a stimulus to community action and involvement.

Existence of any cross-agency forums and networks

In the same way that it is helpful if some community groups already exist in an area, it is also helpful if some formal or informal forums exist in an area linking different local workers and agencies. Again, this is a ready-made resource to tap into if it does exist, and may in turn be a source of information and contacts with local people – for example, health visitors or housing officers may be willing to pass on publicity about the needs assessment to their clients/tenants or even encourage them to get involved. Local workers are likely, collectively, to be able to give a useful overview of what services and resources exist in an area, and to have their own views about local gaps and needs. These should not substitute for getting local people's direct views, as agency priorities and local people's priorities can often differ. However, workers can provide a pool of information to compare and contrast local people's views with, and if similar issues are being raised from both perspectives then an even stronger case can be made for taking action on the needs emerging.

Another reason for involving local workers is to avoid future blocks and barriers; some participatory needs assessment exercises have had their methodology, and thus their findings, rubbished by angry local workers who feel a biased view has been obtained, particularly if there is criticism of local services. However, if workers are involved in the process they are much more likely to see the needs emerging as a way of enhancing local services than as a direct criticism of them, and can be part of a partnership with local people to push for changes and improvements.

Again, as with community groups and networks, a participatory needs assessment can be a stimulus to setting up a 'professional infrastructure' with forums, networks, and so on being one of the outcomes of a needs assessment initiative, even if there was nothing in place to start with.

Past history of research/needs assessment in the area

Some areas, particularly those that are deemed 'deprived', have often already had a number of research projects focused on them in the past. Local people can therefore feel quite justifiably cynical when another 'needs assessment' exercise comes along, which they may feel will lead to no real improvements or changes. This is one reason why organisation development work must also be part of any needs assessment process. It is often worthwhile revisiting past research reports on an area to see what, if anything, has changed, both in terms of the findings and the recommendations. As the case study illustrates, undertaking a new piece of research, even if it has a slightly different focus and is participatory, may not capture local people's support.

Case Study: Co-ordinating existing research and needs (Saltley, Birmingham)

In Saltley, Birmingham, in 1992, the Health Authority and the Healthy Birmingham Project brought in consultants to undertake a health needs assessment, using a community development approach. Through discussion with local people and agencies it was found that ten different reports had been produced in the last ten years by different agencies and very little had changed, with some problems in fact becoming worse. People were quite rightly suspicious and uninterested in getting involved in a health needs assessment. They were much more concerned with why nothing had happened to their views and research findings in the past. As a result of this feedback a report was compiled by the consultants (Labyrinth 1991), pulling together an overview of all the previous studies, and then local people were asked to say what they thought had changed, and which issues still needed addressing. This then formed the basis of a way forward through a joint local community/local agencies community health forum.

Priority given to the area by other agencies

Within any geographical area different agencies are likely to have different boundaries in terms of how they collect data and organise delivery of services. This can make it difficult when trying to pull together statistical and factual information. For example, some statistics will relate to the ward, others may relate to a wider area. The area you are particularly interested in, for example a village or a housing estate, may overlap into two wards, or may be just one part of a larger ward.

Equally some areas may be given particular status or priority by one agency (for example, Health Action Area, Regeneration Area) but that priority may not be shared by all agencies. In the Limeside case study given earlier, the area was prioritised by the NHS organisations, but was a lower priority for the local authority, with several other areas being deemed to be in higher priority need. This can make for great difficulties when trying to take forward action arising from a needs assessment. Thus, where possible it is important to agree with partner agencies on the area to be focused on before getting local people involved, otherwise there may be little chance of multi-agency responses and partnership working at a later stage.

Definition of a 'community'

Local people will themselves have a very clear idea of what they deem as their local area. Some City Challenge and Single Regeneration initiatives have hit problems by having a number of estates or geographical areas under their total remit, and have found that they can only get community involvement if they reduce back down to individual estates or similar sized/ clearly defined areas. A participatory needs assessment relies on people feeling a vested interest and having knowledge of their local area.

In Tunstall, for example (see earlier case study), the ward boundary for Tunstall North was used to define the area to be focused on in the needs assessment, as statistics for both the health and local authority were collected in this way, and the town centre and most of the surrounding area fell within this ward. However, the ward boundary cut out most of a local authority housing estate that all local people considered to be part of Tunstall. Some of the local people and local agencies working on this particular estate did not want it to be left out of the process.

The same issues can arise when focusing on a 'community of interest'. For example, a broad group of people such as 'black and minority ethnic communities' may consist of such diverse ages, gender, cultural backgrounds, and so on that people may not see themselves as a common community of interest; in the HIV/AIDS field there may be real differences between gay men and drug users, for example, who may not feel they have enough in common to define themselves as a 'common community of interest', even though HIV may be an issue for both groups of people.

Communities are usually self-defining, and although it can be difficult for agencies and professionals, local people will inevitably refuse to see their lives in terms of neat categories and labels which fit the ways agencies usually organise professions and services. This is where a degree of flexibility, and also partnership working, can help.

Organisation development

So far we have mainly explored 'reaching out to the community'. However, there is only any point in undertaking a participatory needs assessment if the organisations who purchase and provide services to communities are prepared to act on the needs that emerge from such a process. This has a number of implications for organisation development.

On many occasions organisations race ahead undertaking needs assessments and getting the community involved without having first considered what else is already going on that can be built on, or with no consideration about how the information and ideas are going to be taken forward. Obviously it is not possible to know in advance exactly what will come out of such a process, but it may be necessary to identify financial and/or staff and/or partnership mechanisms with other organisations before embarking on a needs assessment so that there are some mechanisms and resources to draw on once the needs have been identified. If some of this organisational policy development and planning has not taken place then local people may be left feeling that the whole exercise has been a waste of their time and has raised false hopes.

Other chapters will explore organisation development, and strategic mechanisms for involvement, in more detail. The 'critical path to involvement', featured in Chapter 12 is particularly worth referring to before embarking on a participatory needs assessment. A brief case study based on a needs assessment process carried out in the Western Isles of Scotland follows, to give an indication of practical ways of building in organisation development to a participatory needs assessment process.

Case Study: Building in organisation development to the needs assessment process (Western Isles)

The Western Isles Health Board successfully applied for funding, under a Scottish Office primary health care development initiative, to undertake participatory needs assessment within four different communities within the Isles. Outside consultants were brought in to undertake the work. A multi-agency steering group was established to oversee all four needs assessment processes. This group was comprised of reasonably senior people from the health board, NHS trust and local authority. In order to give this group official status, it was made a sub-group of the 'Healthy Islands Partnership', which was itself linked into the joint planning and finance structures for the Isles.

The Steering Group members met approximately once a month during the nine months of the needs assessment process, both to receive feedback on process and to feed in to the next stages. Each of the four areas was allocated a 'key link person' from the health board (all of whom were also on the Steering Group'). This was partly so that the health board could have some in-depth involvement in the process so that in future that learning would remain inside the organisation, and could be called on for other needs assessment exercises. The other reason was to give the process credibility in the eyes of local people in the four areas. There was some cynicism about whether the health board was really committed to the process and to dealing with the findings, so having a board staff member linked to each area helped to make a visible connection to the board's commitment.

Early in the nine-month process a three-hour workshop was held for all the senior decision makers in the key organisations across the Isles. This included senior elected members and appointed members as well as senior officers. Senior-level representatives of agencies such as the Western Isles Enterprise, utilities and professional bodies such as the Chamber of Commerce were also invited along with statutory organisations. The aim of the workshop was to ensure that all agencies were aware of, and committed to, the needs assessment process at the outset and to the methods and approaches that were being used. Many needs assessments have difficulties in connecting to people and decision-making processes at senior levels. It is easy to disown a process when it has got to the report and recommendations stage if this is the first time people claim to have heard about it. Holding such an event on a multi-agency basis can also be useful as it allows agencies to observe each other's commitment, which can be useful if that needs to be raised at a later stage.

Once the four needs assessments had taken place another workshop, of the same length, and with the same multi-agency, senior-level group of participants, was held. This time the purpose was to feed back the findings and to receive the recommendations. Smaller working groups were formed to explore the implications of the recommendations both from single agency and multi-agency perspectives and to put forward some initial ideas about ways of progressing the recommendations and taking forward action.

The Steering Group continued to meet with two levels of responsibility; first to ensure there were continued links with, and feedback to, the four communities; second, to oversee the implementation of the recommendations.

One year after the initial needs assessment work, a two-day training workshop was held, to which many of the key players in the needs assessment process were invited. This was an opportunity to both consolidate the learning, and to look at the process strategically (Labyrinth 1996d).

In summary, the case study indicates that the organisation development part of any needs assessment also needs time, commitment and ongoing involvement. Key things to build in are:

● Multi-agency involvement at both very senior and operational levels.
● A small steering group made up of people who are prepared (and allowed) to put time and skills into the process at both grass-roots and strategic levels.

- Involvement, and commitment of senior decision makers, at an early stage.
- Feedback to both communities and organisations.
- People who are prepared to follow up recommendations for months (and perhaps occasionally years) after the actual needs assessment has taken place and who have a structural mechanism for doing this.
- An opportunity to reflect on both individual and collective learning, and lessons for the future.

Notes

1   North Staffordshire Health Authority, 'A Multi-City Plan on Urban Primary Health Care Systems: Draft Plan of Work 1995/6' (unpublished internal document).
2   Shirley McIver: notes from her input into an NHS Executive Research and Development Conference on consumer-led isues, 1994.

10 A participatory approach to evaluation

Summary

This chapter looks at the difficulties and problems that have been experienced in trying to gain recognition for community development and health (CDH) as a valid activity that can generate real changes and improvements. It then moves on to look at evaluation approaches and methodology suitable for community development and health work. There is also an examination of different evaluations of community health projects that have taken place over the last few years, and an overview of what these studies show us about the effectiveness of CDH work.

Difficulties and dilemmas with evaluating community development

C.N. Anyanwu (1988) describes community development (CD) as a concept

> ... based on the premise that when people are given the opportunity to work out their own problems, they will find solutions that will have a more lasting effect. Hence ... it is not necessarily the physical improvements effected within a community, but principally the changes that have taken place in people themselves, that count as important in the process of community development. [p. 11]

This clearly has far-reaching implications for research and evaluation. Writers such as Anyanwu and Marie-Therese Feuerstein (1988) have promoted the concept of participatory evaluation as a 'method to fit the people', arguing that the use of such methodology means that 'both researcher and researched become partners in the joint venture of human liberation and mobilization' (Anyanwu 1988, p. 12).

However, as they have noted, issues in relation to 'objectivity', 'validity' and 'truth' are often quickly raised when qualitative research is seen to 'offer up findings and insights which will disturb the status quo' (Finch 1986, p. 197), and instead support the 'powerless and poor', challenging the notion that they should 'continue to be judged by others using sets of assumptions and value judgements constructed very largely without their participation' (Feuerstein 1988, p. 16).

Much of the research traditionally undertaken in the broad health field is of a quantitative nature, and usually bases people and projects in the position of 'subject' of research and evaluation rather than active participants. It has been suggested that 'being cast in the technician role by definition gives the researcher a relatively limited amount of control over the kinds of data which are to be generated and the kind of issues which are to be studied' (Finch 1986, p. 199).

It is well-recognised and documented that CD workers historically have viewed evaluation as a funder's tool that usually employs both personnel and methodology that is unsympathetic or inappropriate to CD work. Indeed, it has been used to justify closing down projects on the ground that they are engaged in 'radical' and 'political' work (see, for example, many of the reports from the 1970s Home Office-sponsored Community Development Projects). This legacy of inappropriateness and distrust of evaluation methodologies has led to situations where outside researchers are often presented with statistics and other data that are, in themselves, meaningless in giving a perspective on the real day-to-day empowerment work of community workers and community health projects.

Brinberg and McGrath state that they wrote their book, *Validity and the Research Process* (1985), as a 'reaction to the view of validity as something to be acquired by diligent application of certain techniques' (p. 13). They expand on this further:

> Validity ... is a concept designated an ideal state – to be pursued but not to be attained ... validity is to do with truth, strength and value. The discourse of our field has often been in the tones that seem to imply that validity is a tangible 'resource' , and that by applying appropriate techniques, one has somehow 'won' at the game called research. [p. 13]

But as M. Rein points out, 'claims of value-neutrality in policy research mean that we take the risk of winning objectivity at the cost of usefulness' (quoted in Finch 1986, p. 198).

Outlining the relationship between research and policy Finch notes that:

Qualitative researchers are not simply in the position of having to persuade policy makers that their concept of 'objective' research is a naïve one, but also have to cope with the reality that quantitative methods which provide 'objective research' are exceedingly useful in relation to the daily task of maintaining the status quo ... qualitative research, in contrast, is much more likely to offer up findings and insights which will disturb the status quo, while at the same time the methods employed make it impossible to claim credibility on the grounds of objectivity. [Finch 1986, p. 197]

Two of the key figures involved in the Health Education Authority's community development work at the end of the 1980s (see Chapter 2) wrote a paper for discussion at a UK conference to explore approaches to evaluating 'Health For All' approaches (Adams and Smithies 1993). They examined issues from the perspective of community health practitioners who have experienced a lack of academic support in the UK for participatory approaches to research and evaluation – for example, the Open University review of the HEA's CD work and role was never published and was subject to much delay and criticism from the HEA's research department on a number of grounds including bias and lack of objectivity. They attempted to provide a rationale for the importance of participatory approaches within evaluation, which links evaluation methodology specifically to community development philosophy and methodology.

Adams and Smithies highlight a number of ways in which community participation strategies pose difficulties for evaluation:

● Various actors and interests, sometimes opposing each other, are involved.
● The work is developmental and the outcomes unpredictable.
● Change is taking place constantly.
● Process is integral and needs evaluating as well as outcomes.
● Evaluation methods should mirror the principles of the approach itself.

The authors assert the importance of dealing with these dilemmas in order to carry out research and evaluation that focuses on illuminating the why and how as well as what and how many. In other words, they advocate the use of qualitative as well as quantitative methods. Conventional evaluation methods are often held up to be more 'objective', reliable and valid. This issue of validity is a crucial one when exploring participative approaches to evaluation. In such a process the role of the researcher or evaluator is not as a producer of 'expert' knowledge but as a facilitator whose task is to support the development of the community's own knowledge. However, involving people in evaluating their own work, products and projects is often seen to introduce a 'bias'. There is somehow an endemic suggestion in these allusions to 'bias' that people cannot distance themselves from their own participation sufficiently to make critical appraisals and evaluate what they have achieved, and most significantly, where they need to move forward to next. People active in the 'Community Health Movement' in the UK are only too aware of how often their endeavours to take forward community development practice and principles into evaluation have led to criticisms of the validity of their methodology and data.

Participatory evaluation is not a substitute for more traditional evaluation methods, rather it is a way to ensure that the approach and technology is more appropriate and effective and fits the needs of the people most closely involved in day-to-day community development work. In conclusion, they assert that:

> Evaluation and research within Health For All needs a radical rethink. It should employ the principles of the new public health movement, i.e.

- It should engage with 'participation' as a dynamic in the process of the research and the way communities and the 'researched' receive the research outcomes.
- Equal opportunities policies should be integrated into research methodologies.
- Researchers and evaluators should work in partnership with their 'subjects' to create new methodologies.
- Researchers need to be accountable to their subjects.
- The research process and intended outcomes should aim to contribute to reducing inequalities in health. [Adams and Smithies 1993, p. 70]

What do we mean by evaluation?

It is very important to be clear from the outset why a particular project, strategy or initiative is being evaluated. Having a clear idea of what purpose an evaluation will serve influences the sorts of information that may need to be collected, and the style and methods adopted.

Evaluation needs to be seen within the overall context of a project's development and monitoring. In an article in *Voluntary Voice*, the newsletter of the London Voluntary Service Council, Sandy Merritt (c. 1988) noted that effective evaluation is part of a much wider process that includes:

- Assessment of needs or problems.

- Assessment of available resources.
- Establishment of clear goals or objectives.
- Developing activities or services to meet those goals.
- Collecting data about what you're doing, while you are doing it.
- Reviewing what you're doing to see if you've done what you set out to do.
- Evaluating what you've done to see if needs have been met or problems solved.
- Learning from the experience and applying what you have learnt to future work.

Implementation of all these stages makes good practical sense in any developmental piece of work as well as ensuring that evaluation is situated within the overall context of a project, rather than an 'add-on'.

Who has a stake in the evaluation?

Another major influence on the development of an appropriate evaluation model is the identification of stakeholders. For example:

- Who is the report/outcome of the evaluation for?
- Who is/are the focus of the project work? (i.e. where is change targeted?)
- Who else is affected directly or indirectly?
- Who will be involved in the evaluation?

Resource implications of different approaches

The availability of resources for monitoring and evaluation, the skills available within the project, and the depth and complexity of the evaluation required all affect the choice of model or framework. Some examples of ways people have approached monitoring and evaluation are set out below. Obviously there are resource implications whichever approach is selected, in terms of finance (in the case of bringing in an outside evaluator, for example) and/or time (especially, for example, in self- or assisted evaluation approaches):

- Full time researcher/evaluator attached to individual projects.
- Researcher/evaluator overseeing a series of projects/a wider strategy.
- Researcher/evaluator retained on an occasional basis.
- Researcher/evaluator brought in at a set point (e.g. end of funding period).

- Researcher/evaluator who co-ordinates assisted self-evaluation.
- Self-evaluation.

Some key questions

The following key questions need to be clarified at this early stage:

1   What purpose(s) will an evaluation serve?
2   Who will be the target audience for the evaluation?
3   Who will be involved in the evaluation process?
4   What resources (including time, people, money) are available for monitoring and evaluation?
5   What issues/areas of activity does the project wish to prioritise for evaluation purposes?
6   What 'evidence' would constitute 'success'?
7   How will data and information be collected?
8   How will data and information be analysed and by whom?
9   How will the evaluation be presented; what format(s) are felt to be appropriate?

These may need to be discussed by funders, managers/management committee members, paid staff, volunteers, project users and any other significant individuals and organisations, and a consensus arrived at. Clearly, the sooner decisions can be reached, the sooner a process can be put into place. Too many initiatives struggle with these issues at a stage when the project's funding may be coming to an end, rather than building in evaluation planning at an early stage in the initiative's development.

Community development approaches to evaluation

There are key elements which distinguish community development evaluation from a more traditional model. The methods of evaluation must themselves emphasise the same elements as the CD process itself. That is, in order for evaluation work to follow CD principles it must:

- Form part of a process – That is, it happens in some form throughout the life of the piece of work being evaluated. The findings and results are constantly used to help make appropriate changes and increase effectiveness of the work. It is not something 'tacked on' at the end, but is used as a moulding tool.

- Be participative – Participants in the community development process must be involved at every level of the evaluation, with or without the help of an external facilitator. Thus they are involved in the process of evaluation, rather than seen as simply the raw material to be studied. .

- Facilitate self-evaluation – That is, whether or not an external facilitator or consultant is used, the evaluation must leave the participants with increased skills, knowledge and confidence in actively doing evaluation, as opposed to being evaluated passively.

- Lie within an equalities framework – That is, any evaluation must be sure to ask questions about who is, and who is not, involved in a piece of work, and what methods are used to encourage participation by all appropriate groups.

Case Study: Evaluation lessons for small projects and organisations

The Thamesdown Evaluation Project (TEP) commenced in 1990 (Thamesdown 1994). It was funded for three years to develop local and national understanding of the role of evaluation in small/community organisations, and to enhance the knowledge and skills required to undertake and manage evaluation. A number of lessons were learnt from the work:

- Installing evaluation and learning from the experience is often a long and difficult process, given limited resources within voluntary and community organisations.
- Involving all individuals in an organisation in evaluation is often problematic; this requires sustained effort. Sharing experience widely within the organisation means that the results of evaluation will not be diminished by changes in staff.
- Individuals benefit from involvement in evaluation as much as organisations, for example, through confirmation that their work is valued by users and/or through enhanced communication between parts of an organisation.
- Putting in place ongoing evaluation procedures may take time, and a degree of follow-up may be needed from a project such as TEP.
- Equal opportunities principles can be integrated into the evaluation and its recommendations, but it may take concentrated efforts for small under-resourced organisations to change practices substantially.

TEP also discovered some implications from its work for the development of evaluation support structures:

- Written material alone is only a first stage in the process of evaluation – material needs careful packaging and usually some direct back-up.
- The idea of (ongoing) self-evaluation needs to be instilled in projects.
- Evaluation work can be linked to the needs of funders, with support workers playing an intermediary role.
- A degree of follow-up is almost certainly necessary over time to ensure organisations continue to build on the results of evaluation.
- The need for in-depth work by an external agency will vary depending on the capacity of the organisation.
- Most organisations welcome the use of an external evaluation support worker to provide expertise and objectivity.
- A high degree of initial 'ground work' is needed before an evaluation can be set in place. Therefore, work needs to be managed carefully so that a case load is maintained and efforts with specific projects are pursued over time.
- In establishing a project like TEP, location of the project is important; for example, the problems of legitimacy with funders, maintaining independence and ensuring close contact with local networks are significant factors.

Evaluation models

Marie-Therese Feuerstein (1986) advocates a method of evaluation in which people are involved in defining their own evaluation needs, building on existing intellectual and leadership capabilities and practical skills, and refining group work methods. She has developed an approach to evaluation which uses training to build a common understanding of the meaning and purpose of participatory evaluation among projects. During training the actual evaluation plan is constructed, and a 'core group' of participants assume responsibility for carrying it out within a specific time frame.

In such a process, she argues, the task of the researcher becomes, not to produce knowledge, but to facilitate the construction of knowledge by the community itself. She sees a participatory evaluation approach not only as an evaluative but also an educational approach which, in addition, increases the management capacities of project staff and participants.

The book contains a number of detailed checklists, guidelines and models which will help a facilitator to carry out an evaluation with project participants. These are described under a number of headings:

1 Understanding evaluation.
2 Planning and organising resources.
3 Using existing knowledge and records.
4 Collecting more information.
5 Reporting the results of evaluation.
6 Using your evaluation results.

Of particular use is her description of the evaluation steps:

1 Deciding to evaluate.
2 Choosing evaluation goals and methods. Deciding who will take part, how and when. Making a detailed plan.
3 Collecting materials and resources, beginning the evaluation.
4 Using the evaluation methods chosen, such as questionnaires, surveys, studying records, etc.
5 Studying the facts, figures and information collected during the evaluation.
6 Reaching conclusions, writing them down and studying them.
7 Preparing the report, deciding how to improve monitoring and when to evaluate again.
8 Feedback of results and putting them into practice.

This approach is best envisaged as a circular process rather than a linear set of steps.

In 1992 Gabriel Chanan produced a 'community development monitoring scheme' to help with evaluating the various projects which his organisation, the Community Development Foundation (CDF) were undertaking. The purpose of this scheme was 'to make it easier to report clearly, quickly and regularly on key aspects of community development work' (Chanan 1992). The document includes a set of materials for use by community workers dealing with several different groups or initiatives over a period of time and is geared to a one-year cycle, but can be continued over a number of years. The scheme is intended to reflect a central part of the worker's task, i.e. direct work with community groups and initiatives, but does not reflect the whole of how worker time is spent, nor on the internal processes of the project as a whole. The scheme does not claim to be objective, given that it is based primarily on the worker's perceptions; however, collaboration with community groups in using the materials is also encouraged.

These materials are of particular interest because they attempt to distinguish between the progress of groups and the contributions made by community workers. They also seek to log ideas and potential groups that do not materialise, and to record why they did not develop further. The actual format of the materials is as follows:

- Sheet to undertake initial mapping by setting out the basic profile of each group worked with.
- Sheets to use periodically (every two months is suggested) to record/ analyse work with different groups.
- Sheets to review issues (particularly those relating to specific policy areas) that emerge, as a way of mapping how the interests and activities of different groups connect to each other.
- Format for a one-year report, drawing on all the information recorded through the above materials.

It is suggested that over the year 5 per cent of the community worker's time is spent on recording and analysing developments and progress. It is intended that the materials have a number of uses, including providing fairly detailed records which can be of use in evaluation, in the case of a change of workers, and to assist planning and management of workers and projects.

Evaluating community development and health work

It is worth noting that just as CDH has developed its own infrastructure of networks, resources and publications, so it has developed some specific evaluation approaches. CDH is seen as linked to, though distinct from, general community work and community development. The main differences are in relation to 'stakeholders'. The involvement of NHS agencies and staff is not particularly common in general community work and community development. The emphasis on 'health' means that both aims, practice and monitoring and evaluation may differ. However, most CDH work shares the principles and values of community work, which in turn means that most of the evaluation theory and practice that has been developed is influenced by values/principles such as 'participation', 'empowerment' and 'equity'.

Several key texts are explored below. They have been selected because they give a comprehensive overview of the range of approaches and some of the debates and discussions currently underway in relation to evaluation in the CDH field.

The Open University's review of the CDH work of the Health Education Authority contained a section which focused specifically on evaluation approaches and methodologies (Beattie 1991). It also contained an introduction to terminology, a summary of all available evaluation reports on CD and health between 1979 and 1989, and made comparisons with methodology and evaluation in wider public administration fields and recommendations for improving evaluation strategies.

Several styles of evaluation are identified from a review of the 43 available reports. They are:

- A historical approach; based on an assembled chronological narrative.
- Participatory evaluation; giving priority to the involvement of local people – action research; where the evaluator has a 'hands on' role and ongoing involvement.
- The practitioner as researcher; self-evaluation by the project worker(s).
- The independent external examiner.
- Objectives-based evaluation; systematic checking of progress against set objectives.
- Decision-led evaluation; taking the form of reports, briefing papers etc. – goal-free evaluation; focusing primarily on process.
- Critical view; where a professional judgement is made by an 'expert'.
- Negotiated style; checking data against views and perceptions of key informants.

The variety of tools and techniques used to aid/undertake evaluation are also summarised from the 43 reported examples. These included:

- Work diaries and work records.
- Reports and minutes of meetings.
- Participant observation.
- Questionnaires.
- Interviews, both formal and informal.
- Personal recollections/oral history.
- Group discussion.
- Epidemiological and/or demographic statistical data.
- Outcome indicators.
- Critical incidents/snapshots.
- Case studies.
- Retrospective analysis.
- Prospective studies; starting the evaluation from the outset of a project.

The section concludes:

[N]o one single evaluation method will satisfy or be acceptable to all parties ... there needs to be much more vigorous investment ... in the 'pluralistic' approach. This would seek to build up within a project a 'multi-faceted portfolio' of data and reports, and to ensure a highly active programme of discussion and shared scrutiny of the questions of performance, quality and value that are raised by the project. [Beattie 1991, p. 230]

A final checklist/code of practice for evaluation in relation to CD and health is proposed. It emphasises that any evaluation procedure:

- Should keep rich descriptive records.
- Should ask a few powerful questions.
- Should seek explanations and do essential detective work.
- Must be valid/impartial/objective and/or must make value position clear.
- Must not damage/distort/interfere with the programme (e.g. should be negotiated and collaborative).
- Must have clear rules around confidentiality or disclosure.
- Must offer feedback to project workers/managers for decisions.
- Must be firmly linked to problem solving and remedial action.
- Must be intelligible to external audiences. [Beattie 1991, p. 232]

Evaluators working in the CDH field have sought to take on some of the concerns about developing indicators that can show improvements in health as well as the wider perspectives on improvements in quality of life, outlook, aspirations and changes to services and policies. There has, not surprisingly, been some resistance to the idea of trying to evaluate changes in a person's health – for example, are people less likely to die of a heart attack if a community development and health initiative has been active in the area they live in? – because of the complex nature of the potential factors that influence individual and collective health status. Also, most community health initiatives are small in scale, and operate only for a limited period of time. Any health impact, even if it can be identified and associated directly with community health work, may not show up for many years into the future.

However, one health project did attempt to set out criteria to evaluate its impact on the heart health of the local residents of the area within which the project was based.

Case Study: Evaluating health outcomes from a community health project ('Heart Of Our City', Sheffield)

The Sheffield-based 'Heart of Our City' (HOOC) initiative was one of the longest established action research projects which attempts to link community development approaches with a specific health topic focus (prevention of coronary heart disease), within a specific geographical locality. The project had a full-time research post as part of the staffing resource.

The funding proposal document sets out the proposed evaluation model:

> [T]he essential feature of an evaluation exercise is that it should generate as much usable information as possible ... we have attempted to identify what would be useful information for various groups of stakeholders. Undoubtedly most would be interested in both the process and outcome information of a quantitative and qualitative nature. [Sheffield District Health Authority 1988]

They go on to say that evaluating programmes with a community development approach requires a multi-dimensional strategy utilising a range of research methods.

Examples of qualitative indices for assessing the impact of HOOC, and specific outcomes, drawn from the overall project aims, are set out:

- 25 per cent reduction in premature mortality rate for CHD – to be measured through, for example, monitoring hospital admissions for CHD from the HOOC area, changes in mean population blood pressure.
- Health-related behaviour and lifestyle, through, for example, monitoring the percentage of regular smokers, the percentage who regularly exercise.

However, what is also very important is the emphasis placed on the process indices and measurements, and the project's whole approach to community involvement in monitoring and evaluation. Examples of key questions within the HOOC process evaluation criteria include:

- What mechanisms have been developed for the involvement of the community in the programme's activities?
- What mechanisms have been developed for the involvement of the community in the programme's management?
- What changes and developments in these areas occur throughout the life of the project – and why?

Comparative analysis with other parts of Sheffield, national data, and data from other projects undertaking a community development approach to heart health is part of the overall approach in an attempt to assess to what extent the changes and developments could be specifically attributed to the HOOC project.

A paper exploring key values for HOOC research and evaluation sets out how these will be practically implemented:

> Research within community development must incorporate key values of equity, empowerment, participation and operate within a social framework ... Participation by local people in community development research is of course essential. Ideally participation should mean involvement in the research process from the inception of ideas to data analysis and report writing. (Moody 1992)

The paper goes on to explain how local people have been involved in the initial data collection on which to establish the project's baseline information and to set initial priorities. Future ideas on ways local people could remain involved in the research, monitoring and evaluation processes are also briefly explored. These include:

- Involvement in dissemination of initial findings.
- Oral history work.
- Involvement in surveys of availability of 'healthy' foods in local shops.

The project's research and evaluation process has concluded and findings are available from Sheffield Health Authority and the Health Education Authority.

Case Study: Developing a framework for evaluating a local community health project (Impact 3, North Derbyshire)

Some community health workers, frustrated by lack of funding for outside research and evaluation of their projects, and knowing that their projects were time limited and therefore it was down to them to show the positive impact of their work, have developed their own evaluation frameworks. One such framework is explored below (Rawson and Macredie, undated). It has also been made available to other community health initiatives.

The introduction addresses a number of key questions:

- Why evaluate?

- What should be evaluated?
- Who should do the evaluation?
- When should it be done?
- How will the evaluation be presented?
- What possible implications might there be for the key people and organisations within the project as a result of the evaluation?

A number of responses are then set out to the question 'why evaluate?' This is followed by a breakdown of 'what should be evaluated?' The process and outcomes of the following are identified as main areas for the evaluation to focus on:

- Management structure.
- Worker and community support.
- Contact with workers (range, purpose and quality of ...).
- Contact with communities (range, purpose and quality of ...).
- Effectiveness of groups.
- Training set up for workers; community groups; individuals.
- Collaborative work.

Different people are then identified as being responsible for evaluating within the different categories set out above (this will obviously vary from project to project). The Community Development Worker features in all seven categories; project managers, local people, local groups, local workers and trainers and participants feature in relation to specific relevant categories.

Timescales for how often each part of the evaluation will be undertaken are highlighted; again, these vary between two-monthly to annually, depending on the area of focus.

Methods to undertake the evaluation also vary depending on the focus, and who is involved. They include:

- Short proformas.
- Longer questionnaires.
- Verbal feedback.
- Baseline survey/interviews.
- Photographs.
- News clippings.
- Tape recordings.
- Leaflets.
- Posters.
- Write-ups.

The importance of demonstrating benefits to local communities is given particular attention. The following are used:

- Feedback from groups about what they think they have gained.
- Levels of activity: number of groups; range of work.
- Development of infrastructure.
- Workers.
- Groups.

The report then moves on to set out in some detail how ongoing work, such as networking, identifying community health needs, working with groups, working with workers' support mechanisms, and training, fit in with the evaluation protocol. It ends with examples of the sorts of questions that can be built in to the different evaluation approaches and areas of focus. The questions are divided into three main types: process, quantitative and qualitative.

Examples of *process*-type questions include: Did activities lead to desired outcomes, changes sought and objectives initially built into the project? Did activities represent good uses of resources, particularly time?

Examples of *quantitative* questions include: How many people attended activity? Which groups of the community did they represent?

Examples of *qualitative* questions include: What was the quality of the participation? How did people feel about the activity?

The evaluation protocol explored above forms the structure for the actual evaluation report undertaken at the end of Year 2 of the Impact 3 project, i.e. April 1996 (Rawson and Macredie 1996).

What do recent evaluations tell us about CDH work and evaluation approaches?

A recent report (Labyrinth 1996f) looked at eight evaluation reports focusing on seven small locally-based community development and health projects. Since the demise of the National Community Health Resource (NCHR) a few years ago, there is no one place in this country that logs and stores evaluations of this kind. As many of the reports are written for local use they cannot usually be tracked down by a database search at a library; most have never been formally published.

The projects were:

- Impact 3 Community Health Project: North Derbyshire.
- Ince Community Health Project: Wigan.
- Hutson Street Health Project: Bradford (two separate evaluations three years apart).
- Limeside Health Partnership: Oldham.
- Riverside Community Health Project: Newcastle upon Tyne.
- CHOICE Project: Corby.
- Heeley Health Project: Sheffield.

The seven projects featured had a number of things in common:

- A community development approach is explicit.
- The projects all work within a given local area (though the projects also get involved in City/Town-wide work sometimes).
- All the projects are based in areas which are deemed to be 'deprived' in some sense (rural and urban perspectives are slightly different in this respect).
- All the projects are/have been subject to time-limited funding.
- All the projects are focusing on health in its widest sense (although there are some contradictions in the case of the CHOICE Project in relation to its aims and the focus of some aspects of its evaluation).
- All the projects link directly or indirectly (Hutson Street via Joint Finance) into health authorities and/or trusts.

All of these projects have been formally evaluated. This is not necessarily always the case. There are a lot more community development and health initiatives in existence than evaluation reports!

Of the eight evaluations, six (Ince, Riverside, CHOICE, Heeley and Hutson Street – both evaluations) used outside evaluators; two (Limeside and Impact 3) relied predominantly on the project worker for co-ordinating and carrying out the evaluation. Outside evaluators came from universities in four cases, and from independent consultancy organisations/individuals in two (Ince and the second Hutson Street report).

Of the five projects who brought in external evaluators, three (Ince, the second Hutson Street Project and CHOICE) brought them in towards the end of the project's funding. The first Hutson Street evaluator was linked to the project for its first three years of funding. The remaining two projects produced evaluation reports at interim stages in their existence.

There are a few similarities in the style of the evaluation reports. Most begin with some overview of the project's history and background, and set out the methods used in the evaluation. However, after that there is little in common.

The Ince, Riverside, the second Hutson Street and Limeside evaluations give the most specific detail about the impact of the projects at a variety of levels, for example, local people, local workers, agencies. CHOICE and the first Hutson Street report are most concerned with the general lessons that can be learnt, and with an analysis of the community development process as it relates to health. Impact 3 and Heeley are interim evaluation reports, and as such are primarily concerned with recording what has gone on to date, and looking generally towards the next stages of the project.

It is difficult to make overall comparisons between the seven projects (of course they were never set up to be compared and so there are no common criteria in operation). However, the main thing the evaluations do have in common is that, overall, they come out positively in favour of community development approaches to health. Even in the case of the CHOICE Project, which seems to have run into a number of problems and difficulties, the evaluators are more critical of the way the project was set up and managed than the community development approach as such.

None of the evaluations tries to compare the impact of the community development projects with use of the same level of funding for other types of workers (e.g. health visitors) or approaches in a local area. However, what is consistently highlighted are ways that such projects can enhance the working together and sharing of information between different workers and agencies in a local area. It seems that the projects also harness the involvement of other local workers and agencies, as well as local people, in order both to improve services and support for local people and to maximise the impact of their own small teams (or individual workers in four cases).

Only three of the evaluations (INCE, the second Hutson Street Project and CHOICE) make specific attempts to look at the explicit health (in the medical sense) impact of the projects on local people. However, all the projects and/or evaluators make clear that a broad definition of health is being used; thus the impact of such projects is likely to be very wide-ranging and long-term, as well as having some short-term effects.

The scale of the projects (usually engaging one worker, occasionally a small team) has to be taken into account when looking at outcomes. Many community health projects have aims that are grander than those of the whole of the NHS, with its large budget and staffing resources. Most of the projects featured here have aims which are about process; outcomes are related to changes that can be more realistically achieved and measured, such as increasing people's awareness of health issues, increasing access to health information, etc. Logically this should potentially improve people's health, but this has to be looked at within the broader context of socio-economic factors and other effects on people's health, such as levels of pollution, quality and quantity of local services, etc. There are no known evaluation studies that have been sufficiently resourced to take on such a complex, long-term evaluation approach.

What the evaluation reports do all show (with the slight exception of CHOICE) is that local people value the projects, and enjoy participating in the events, groups and activities. Individuals certainly make clear the impact they feel such projects have on their confidence, enjoyment and sense of involvement in their community life.

In order that readers can get a feel of different approaches taken to evaluating CDH projects, three further case studies follow, which summarise both the approaches taken by the evaluators, and some of their findings. All three are more detailed looks at evaluations mentioned above. Interestingly the Riverside project, which is the subject of the first case study, is one of the longest established (perhaps even the longest) community health projects in the UK.

Case Study: Evaluation of Riverside Community Health Project (Newcastle upon Tyne)

This summary is based on one of three reports produced by researchers from the University of Northumbria that focus on the Riverside Community Health Project in the Benwell area of Newcastle upon Tyne. One report logs the history of the project; another report explores the links between health, poverty and community; this report looks at the outcomes of the project's work (Green and Price 1996).

The project, a locally managed voluntary sector organisation, was initially known as the Riverside Child Health Project, and was both one of the earliest such projects established in the UK and also one of the most long-lasting. The present project came about in 1991 and the evaluation was initiated three-and-a-half years into its new life. The main fieldwork was carried out between October 1994 and April 1995.

This report initially sets out the context for the evaluation by looking at 'Why evaluate?' The main purpose of the evaluation is said to be

> ... to enable those with a stake in the Project – staff, management committee, users, workers from other agencies, funders – to make informed judgements as to the worth and value of its policies and activities. [Green and Price 1996, p. 3]

The methodology used was participatory and the intention was that this would contribute to the ongoing development of the project's work. The report then moves on to look at 'What is a Community Health Project?' This section notes:

> Despite the plethora of statistical studies ... there is still little known about the detailed experience of living in poverty, and in particular of its health effects. Small community-based projects like Riverside represent a unique opportunity for access to the experiences of families raising children on low incomes in difficult social conditions.
>
> ... The primary focus of the Riverside Project is on child health, but this is within an understanding that child health needs are most appropriately addressed through a holistic approach which sees these needs within the context of the family, the community and the wider society. [p. 5]

The main part of the report describes the actual work of the project. Analysis of the work programme suggested breaking it down into eight key categories, each of which includes a case study, as well as detailed description. The categories are:

- Running a local community facility.
- Community and social support.
- Organising groups and activities for local people.
- Facilitating community-based and inter-agency work.
- Community development.
- Influencing policy and practice.
- Contributing to major policy development.
- Research and information collecting.

An analysis of which local people, and which agencies, the project works with is included. The report notes:

> The Riverside Project works, in different ways, with large numbers of people from different neighbourhoods, social groups, and ethnic backgrounds. It is not possible to quote a single figure for the number of people worked with, partly because the Project does not comprehensively monitor its activities in terms of quantitative measures – but more importantly because the complex nature of its work would render such a measure meaningless. [p. 24]

The researchers noted that the project worked mainly, but not exclusively, with women: 'This, however, is not a result of targeting, but is a reflection of a situation whereby women tend to represent the majority of community activists at the neighbourhood level' (p. 24). The project has also successfully targeted ethnic minority families. The section that considers which agencies the project works with notes that the project was seen as having a key role in relation to joint working and makes a major contribution through co-ordination, leadership and support: 'The Project's main strengths were seen by others as flowing from its long term and continuous involvement in the neighbourhood and in health work. Its independence was also seen as a source of strength' (p. 26).

The report concludes that different people see Riverside in different ways, depending on their levels of involvement and reasons for interacting with the project. The 46 different agencies and local people who participated in evaluation produced a set of complex issues of the project, which are illustrated by a series of direct quotes.

The researchers do not try to simplify the impact of the project by looking at it in isolation, but rather include a section which puts Riverside's work within the wider local and national context of changes and challenges, such as unemployment, mounting social problems, changes in the ways health and community care services are organised and delivered, and the emergence of regeneration initiatives.

Within this wider complex picture the report notes:

> There is encouraging evidence that Riverside's contribution to health and social services priorities is increasingly being recognised within the statutory sector ... Riverside works directly or indirectly with thousands of local people in West Newcastle. Its impact is demonstrable, if not always measurable in quantitative terms. [p. 31]

The main findings of the evaluation, in terms of the success of the project's work are:

- The importance of the longevity, stability and embeddedness in the local community.
- The apparently routine and unremarkable work at grassroots level that provides the project and other agencies with an invaluable network of contacts and local knowledge.
- The ability to involve local people and to act as a source of a valuable critical perspective in relation to the practices and policies of the statutory sector.
- The project's unique role in elucidating the wider health consequences of the growing social divisions resulting from economic changes and social policies.

Some of the 'findings' that arose during the evaluation were immediately acted on and addressed because of the participatory nature of the methodology. However, five outstanding key points were identified for the project to address. These are:

- Priority to be given to an unobtrusive but effective system of monitoring and the development of indicators for measuring its effectiveness.
- Improvements made in the ways that the project documents and disseminates its experience and knowledge.
- Development of a more explicit role in investigating and illustrating the relationship between health and poverty, and keeping this on the policy agenda.
- Review its mechanisms for local and user accountability, in relation to empowerment of local people.
- Review its systems for communication and contacts with health services staff.

Case Study: Evaluation of the 'Choice' Project, Corby

This case study (Luck and Jesson 1995) summarises an evaluation of the Corby CHOICE Project, which operated from 1989 for three years. CHOICE is an acronym based on Choose Healthy Option in Corby Everyday. It was funded as one of three initiatives selected by the Oxfordshire Regional Health Authority and contracted through the Kettering Health Authority. The evaluation began in 1992 and was undertaken by researchers from Aston Business School.

The report starts with the rationale for the evaluation and the background to the CHOICE Project. It then moves on to put the methodology used for this particular evaluation into the wider context of community health development evaluation.

The definition of community health development used (p. 7) is based on a quote from a paper written by Lee Adams in 1989:

> Community Development of Health encompasses a commitment to a holistic approach to health which recognises the central importance of social support and social networks. A community development way of working attempts to facilitate individual and collective action around common needs and concerns. These concerns and needs are identified by people themselves, rather than being imposed from outside.

The concept of 'community' is also explored, along with the history and ideology of community development. Evaluation of community health development is said to often present dilemmas and conflict in terms of methodology:

In health projects conflict arises because the community development objectives, of increasing self confidence, promoting better relationships and extending public influence, have outcomes which can rarely be measured in quantitative terms (of epidemiology, morbidity, mortality) that the funders can recognise. [p. 13]

The researchers also go on to note that there are a number of features intrinsic to community health development projects which make them difficult to evaluate. These are:

- their relative newness;
- their relative unconventionality;
- most objectives and priorities change, because events are in a continuing process (outcomes rarely match objectives);
- there are few tangible measurable outcomes (it is difficult to measure changes in behaviour which will have long term effects); and
- there is no control group. [p. 16]

The methodology actually chosen for the evaluation of the CHOICE Project was process evaluation which involved the evaluators becoming 'participant observers'. They also drew on the results of an initial lifestyle survey undertaken at the outset of the project, a small number of *ad hoc* surveys and the interim review of the project's activities.

The lifestyle survey follow-up indicated that there had been improvements in terms of three factors:

- a shift from full fat to semi-skimmed milk;
- a reduction in total amount of alcohol drunk especially by heavy drinkers; and
- an increase in ex-smokers. [p. 23]

The report's authors note that it is difficult to associate these changes specifically with the CHOICE Project, as there have been no controls for other variables that effect the health of local people in an area, and also the lack of relevant local statistical information. Although the before and after lifestyle survey work was seen, in the funding proposal, as the main means of evaluating success, community development methodology was not adopted until after the funding application had been successful. Thus the evaluation methodology and focus was no longer as appropriate.

The interim review of project activities was carried out about half-way through the life of the project. This was an attempt to build up a picture of the project, and what had shaped its work and practice. Charts which map

192 Community Involvement in Health

and analyse the work are reproduced in this evaluation report. The main conclusions of this review were:

- the Kingswood estate had limited sense of community and it was difficult for the CHOICE workers to involve residents in CDH activities;
- local health workers were antagonistic to CHOICE;
- there had been some success in drawing in local authority workers and resources into Kingswood; and
- the CHOICE workers were not working as a team and they had tended to deal with inter-personal and conceptual difficulties by working separately. [p. 19]

The ways in which the four workers were recruited into the team, and the lack of a clear management structure, were identified as limiting factors on the effectiveness of the work. Conflicts of personalities and aims arose from the lack of cohesion in terms of methods of recruitment and broad combination of background experiences and skills. Work undertaken by the different team members is described as 'disparate and lacking focus'.

The evaluators worked with women from a local community group, established by the CHOICE Project to undertake a 'Resident's Impact Survey'. Of the 250 residents interviewed, only 30 per cent had ever heard of any of the project's activities. However, some people named activities that had begun in the area, without associating them with CHOICE.

The goal of CHOICE was to help residents think about making healthy choices, and most of those who had heard of the project recognised that aim and understood the nature of the work. About half of those who had heard of CHOICE had been involved in the project's activities. This section of the report concludes:

On the whole only a minority of people felt that CHOICE had actually been successful and they were critical of the low level of publicity, but those who had benefited spoke of improved facilities, new group activities, improved community participation and improved healthy outlook. [p. 21]

A 'Professionals Impact Survey' was also undertaken. The majority of those interviewed (six months after the completion of the CHOICE Project) expressed very positive views about the project and the workers. Cost effectiveness of this way of working was raised by a minority of critical professionals. One encouraging outcome was that over half of the organisations represented in the sample said that CHOICE had made a difference to their own organisations and the way that health promotion was perceived.

Within this sample, however, health service staff were the least likely to say that their organisation had changed or were going to take community development as a health promotion approach in the future. The evaluators note:

> Looking back, it would have been more useful if the process evaluation had been carried out earlier, and the CDH principles had been made explicit and agreed by all the workers, and had been repeated at regular intervals throughout the project. [p. 27]

However, they were able to draw out some lessons from the evaluation, including:

- The need to consider evaluation from the outset, and include funds for outside evaluation in community health project budgets as well as building it into workers' job descriptions.
- More consideration of the make-up of skills and expertise in the team, and support for cohesive team working to common aims.
- The need for a suitable local base.
- The need for a clear line management structure within the project team.
- The need for clear messages to other local health workers about the role and responsibilities of community development workers, and some attempt to work in partnership and offer complementary support to local people.

The report has three final conclusions:

1 There should be careful preparation with local professionals and residents before the project begins, so that tensions can be anticipated and worked through.
2 There should be a firm management structure to the project with clear lines of accountability including responsibility to the community.
3 In order to overcome the limitations of short term projects, long term funding is needed [pp. 27–28].

Case Study: Evaluation of Heeley Health Project, Sheffield

This evaluation (Ritchie 1992) is based on the first 18 months of the Heeley Health Project; the project is still in existence to date, the Community Operational Research Unit (CORU) evaluator stayed actively involved in the project, but no further reports have yet been produced.

The report starts by summarising the background of the project and notes that CORU were approached at an early stage to help support the development of an evaluation model and to undertake the evaluation as an outside organisation. Discussions with the management committee and the project community development worker concluded that a 'portfolio approach' to evaluation should be adopted, i.e. a range of methods for recording, presenting and analysing activities: 'To this end, the Project has created a record of the Project including diaries and photographs and quantitative and qualitative information based on questionnaires, observation and interviews' (p. 1).

The report notes that the project is based on community development principles and as such the events and groups that have been established are as a result of community consultation. The project has also been involved in some city-wide work as well as neighbourhood initiatives.

This evaluation is primarily intended for 'internal' use, i.e. for the management committee, worker and project users, rather than to justify the project to outside agencies:

> No attempt has been made to establish 'control groups' or to undertake strict 'scientific' monitoring of activities and their impact. These were felt to be neither appropriate nor possible within the working practices or resources available to the Project. [p. 1]

When looking to the evaluation of the project in the future the writer of this report notes:

> It is necessary to be realistic about the level of evaluation that the Project could – and indeed SHOULD – undertake. The Project will inevitably be one amongst many factors affecting the local health picture. The management committee must seriously consider what level of resources would be needed in order to undertake a more broad ranging evaluation which would focus on the impact of the Project on the 'health of Heeley as a whole'. There are also serious ethical problems in extending the evaluation to focus on individuals which could seriously compromise the style of working of the Project. [p. 2]

At the point that this report was written the project was to embark on a major community health profile involving groups and individuals within the community as well as analysis of statistical data already available. It is suggested that the findings of the profile could inform future evaluation activities.

The methodology used for this first stage of evaluation is Systems Resource evaluation, which relies on an 'expert' judging the performance of an organisation against a number of systems characteristics. These are drawn from a broad list of 'critical characteristics of a health system', and applied, in the form of a series of specific questions, to this particular project. There are seven in all. These are:

1   Does the project have aim(s)?
2   Is the project able to monitor what is happening in Heeley (and beyond) and to communicate appropriately?
3   Is the project able to use information to make policy?
4   Is the project able to ensure that policy is carried out?
5   Is the project able to secure the necessary resources?
6   Is there sufficient and appropriate communication within the project?
7   Does the project operate the appropriate levels of control and independence – of groups and worker(s)?

The evaluator documents and reflects on activity and evidence under each of the questions, and then concludes that the project seems to satisfy most of the systems criteria, and so therefore has the capacity to be a successful project, i.e. is viable.

The report goes on to log the activities developed and undertaken by the project. Groups and courses are focused on initially. Some of the information is quantitative (e.g. 107 different people have been involved in groups or courses set up by the project); where people live in relation to the project; the gender make-up of the different groups and courses, and the total numbers of participants in each event/course are also recorded.

Qualitative information, based on interviews with group members is also included. Three groups – Herbal Health, Food Issues Group, and Agewell – were interviewed by the evaluator. The following quotes give an idea of how the groups are working.

Herbal Health

The feeling was that those who had initially come along 'just out of interest' had now dropped out and attendance at the group remained high, with 10–12 out of the 15 regularly attending. There was a positive feeling that it was important to work in groups rather than the traditional teacher/student role. There was also an enthusiasm to meet and work with members of other groups associated with the Project. There was also a feeling that the attachment to the Project prevented the group from becoming 'too middle class'. [p. 12]

Food Issues Group

The group started with an educational feel about it – because that is what the original members had wanted – but had now moved onto a more campaigning basis.

There had been quite a high turnover in the group, possibly because some people had been interested mainly in the educational aspects. There was a feeling that the group was now too small and that members of the group needed to make positive attempts at recruitment.

However, the current members were enthusiastic – particularly about the prospect of the food audit, which they were about to undertake. They felt that there was a real opportunity to influence local shops. [p. 12]

Agewell

The main reason that most people had become involved was to meet people, have a chat and a cup of tea. The health focus was incidental. However, having joined there was a real interest in health issues which prevented the group from becoming a social club or just another meeting place. Most of the group lived alone and a major benefit of their involvement was meeting people in the street and having a chat with them. However, the group was seen as more focused than this and it was strongly felt that the health theme was important.

The group clearly valued their own worth – they weren't prepared to be dismissed or sidelined just because they were old. They were very positive about sharing their skills and crafts with each other, as well as learning and doing new things.

The group is likely to become more self managing and undertake organisation of events and trips, but they are likely to continue to need support. [p. 13]

The four main events the project has been involved in are also analysed. These events were:

- Information and activities day.
- Performance and discussion about NHS changes.
- Play about breast cancer, with discussion afterwards.
- Activities for women to try out.

The author noted: 'Comments indicated that the events are viewed as both entertaining and informative. Clearly these types of events have an important role within the overall activities of the Project' [p. 14].

The evaluator then moves on to look at where the project fits into the neighbourhood as a whole. Interviews were undertaken with five people working in the local area for other organisations, to get their perspective on the project's work and impact. The following emerged from these discussions:

- The project had carefully fitted in with existing structures and activities in the area.
- The project was seen as flexible and versatile, with a broad view of health.
- The project had helped turn ideas into action, e.g. establishment of a community shop, and was felt to be a practical resource.
- The project's connection with a local centre and surgery (physically based in same building) was felt to be useful, but the fact that the project also used other bases in the community for groups and activities was felt to be important.
- The existence of the project had clearly attracted additional health related resources into the area.
- The project's potential to involve a wider group of health professionals in community activities was highlighted.
- People wondered whether or not the project was managing to involve people who are not particularly articulate or well-motivated.

The final part of the report takes all eleven of the project's aims, and discussed the project's success in achieving each aim. This allows the evaluator to both reflect and draw on evidence and examples from earlier sections of the evaluation. In summary, it was found that:

- Some local people have been encouraged to identify and express their health needs and concerns.
- Awareness of health inequalities has heightened to some extent.
- Increased knowledge about the preventable nature of many diseases, and the range of ways people can become involved in health in their communities have been addressed in practical ways.
- Enabling individuals to access information and make positive and informed choices has been addressed, and there are ways this could be taken forward further.
- Helping individuals to develop their confidence and take more control over their lives was felt to have been a focus of all the events and groups.
- Involving local people in the management of the project was an aim

that had not yet been met, though steps to move this forward were in hand.

- Work to address discrimination and promote positive action towards disadvantaged groups was difficult to assess as close monitoring had not been undertaken. However, activities with women, older people and people with disabilities all featured high in the project's profile.
- Development of appropriate methods of evaluation and monitoring was being addressed both by the production of this report and by a review of methods after this report was written.
- The final aim, which was to learn from the development process and seek to establish the project in the longer term, was being addressed by various funding proposals (and as we have the benefit of hindsight and know they were successful, then we also know that this aim has been achieved).

11 Management of change

Summary

This chapter begins by looking at definitions of change management and organisation development and moves on to look at the connections between community development and change. A case study is used to look at how one health organisation is trying to take forward community development by taking a strategic organisation development approach to managing large-scale change, in terms of the way its staff and structures relate to local service users, communities and the voluntary sector. The links between community development and organisation development are explored in terms of both stages in the process, and levels of intervention. This theme is further developed to look at different levels of change in terms of health, ranging from individual changes in lifestyles through to national and international policies. Finally the chapter explores a range of change management tools and techniques which can be used with community groups, teams and organisations to help manage change.

Definitions

Mention has been made in many of the previous chapters of organisation development (OD) and change management. The term 'organisation development' is often used loosely to mean any changes and developments that an organisation goes through – be they imposed through outside pressures and initiatives or initiated internally. However, there is also a professional discipline of OD with its own professional association (the International

199

Registry of Organization Development and Professionals). It is still predominantly a way of working which is recognised and used within the private sector, but OD is starting to creep slowly into the public sector. For instance, management of change has become a feature of the work done by the NHS Training Division (see, Caple 1990; Pedlar and Boutall 1992). Some NHS organisations now employ internal OD consultants/officers, as do some local authorities. Most employ outside consultants on short or longer-term projects concerned with helping them to 'manage change'.

Managing change has been defined as:

- Taking control.
- Shaping the direction.
- Influencing the outcome of change.

Management is focused on two parallel strategies and tactical plans: *what* you want to change and *how* you intend to implement change.

Equal weight is given to implementing change, i.e. how to actually go about the process of bringing about the conditions for effecting change, how to get people to commit to change and to stay involved (Plant 1987). Organisation Development (OD) has been described as:

> ... an holistic approach to working with organisations that attempts to link the issues of external adaptation (what is [sic] the responses to outside world) and internal integration (how does the organisation best structure itself to achieve its aims). OD seeks to ensure that both the formal (structures, constitutions, rules and policies) and the informal (values, assumptions, feelings) aspects of organisations are linked to ensure organisational effectiveness.[1]

Community development and change

Effective community development and health work clearly needs to involve change. Change may be at four separate but linked levels.

Individual change may occur through the increased skills, knowledge, confidence and opportunities opened up to people when they are involved in community development and health work. Evaluation reports and personal involvement in CDH work indicates that some people who get actively involved in community activity go on to undertake further education and training and/or gain employment; many people have an increased understanding of how organisations such as the local authority work, how decisions are made and how to push for change. These changes can range from individual concerns such as changing a GP to wider local issues such

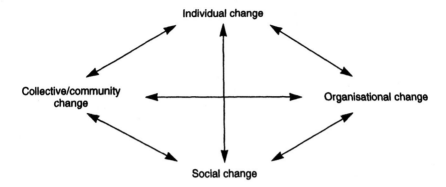

Individual change

Collective/community change

Organisational change

Social change

Figure 11.1   Levels of change in community development and health work

as getting changes in service provision as people feel they know more about health issues for themselves and their families (Kilminster 1996; Labyrinth 1996f).

The NHS is usually concerned with influencing people's individual lifestyle choices and behaviour (e.g. smoking, exercise, etc.) but such changes usually come about as part of a much wider change in attitudes, income levels and social and economic opportunities. However, some evaluation reports have indicated that people do make changes in their lifestyles as a result of involvement with community health projects (Kilminster 1996; Labyrinth 1996f).

Collective/community change is concerned with changes that move beyond benefiting individuals and affect a whole geographical community or at least part of that community. Examples such as campaigns for road crossings, the establishment of play groups or a toy library, or improvements to a bus service are all concerned with changes which affect some or all of a community. Many community initiatives undertaken by the public sector are concerned with generating this sort of collective change. In many cases this is based on a combination of community needs and aspirations and targets set by local and national agencies.

For example, many regeneration initiatives are concerned with increasing employment and improving the social and economic fabric of specific communities. Although many communities share these concerns they may also have their own priorities – for example in relation to crime, housing, youth activities, etc. Most regeneration initiatives now recognise in both their funding bid and implementation stages that a partnership with local communities to set priorities is vital if real change is to occur (Department of the Environment 1997b).

Organisational change is concerned with developments in relation to the organisations and agencies which work in a community, or provide services and support to specific communities of interest, most of which will also have wider district/city/county-wide responsibilities. In order to facilitate some of the individual and collective changes outlined above it may be necessary to make changes at different levels within organisations. For example, one of the needs assessment exercises in the Western Isles of Scotland (Labyrinth 1996g) indicated that a particular service (in this case, physiotherapy) was not performing well, based on feedback from local people. This gave the health purchasers the opportunity to renegotiate the contract they had with the health provider. Wider-scale organisational change may also be needed if there are to be real partnerships between public sector organisations and staff and local people. Changes might be in relation to attitudes, skills, times and places that services are delivered, changes in roles and responsibilities, even the culture and priorities of organisations.

One NHS Trust has taken seriously the challenges implicit in moving towards being a community development-oriented organisation and is at the early stages of a very sophisticated, ambitious change management programme. It is set out below as a case study.

Case Study: An organisation development approach within one NHS organisation[2]

Type of organisation: NHS (Combined Healthcare) Trust
Size of organisation: 3,500 staff

Impetus for Organisation Development: Chief Executive wanted to build an organisation committed to and working for community involvement at every level.

Starting point: Series of five workshops for 50 selected staff (managers and others interested) to look at 'managing change'.

What happened at the workshops:

- Initial enthusiasm.
- Distress and suspicion about what was behind it – fear of possible redundancies.
- Chief Executive came clear about his vision for an organisation with CD central to all its policies and practices – inspired people.

- Dejection about *how* to change the organisation appropriately, given the NHS purchaser/provider split; limited resources; size of the organisation; high numbers of clinically trained staff to whom CD is maybe anathema.
- Practical ideas for first steps in bringing about change.
- Agreement about need for co-ordination and for most of the group to continue with some level of involvement in the change process.

Taking forward the 'how': Secondment of key manager to head up a new unit as 'Director of Learning and Change', with staff of two from old Training and Development Section, plus one new appointment focusing on CD/partnership building with local groups and the voluntary sector.

Action so far:

- Trust has signed up for 'Investors in People' – so all staff feel valued as their commitment to the changes is crucial.
- Project management training offered to all the initial 50 people, plus others who are interested – so all staff can play a role in taking forward action, whatever their formal role and level in the organisation, and so all follow the same process, whatever the project: leading to the creation of virtual teams for one-off projects.
- Induction – improved system set up so all new staff attend an induction day [held weekly] – so all get the message about the importance of CD.
- Organisation of regular inter-agency seminars – range of topics, all with a community focus.
- Lifelong learning initiative (funded by TEC) – for all staff to do any 'learning' in own time, not work-related – emphasises importance of learning and change to the organisation.
- Roadshows comprising displays, discussions, workshops, staff feedback of ideas – presented to all premises and staff by the 50 key players setting out the vision of a CD-led organisation.
- Voluntary sector partnerships – formal links established between a range of voluntary organisations and non-executive members of Board – gives them a role and a relationship to voluntary sector activity.
- Aiming high – inter-agency project to help young people 'aim high' – Trust involved in this along with other partner agencies – gives the organisation visibility both as a potential employer and service provider to young people.
- Development of a corporate set of 'qualities' in relation to CD – used as part of each member of staff's personal review.

- Development of international links – to help staff see other ways of working and delivering services in partnership with communities – staff are selected for study visits to other countries, and then feedback to others to expand the vision of what can be done.
- Large-scale reorganisation to look at a locality-based structure for the organisation as opposed to specialist area-type structure to allow for more cross-disciplinary working and linking more closely to local areas and people.
- Multi-skilling training, i.e. expanding some people's jobs so they can more effectively cross role and organisational boundaries.
- Collaborative care planning – encourage team working.
- Staff involvement in a successful local Single Regeneration Bid area – direct links and partnerships with communities and other agencies to bring about change.
- Management bonus – to spend on involvement in a learning programme or materials.
- OD support offered to different parts of the organisation, e.g. to facilitate team working in wards.

Levels of change

The organisation featured in the case study above would be the first to admit that it has a long way to go in its change process and that there are many hurdles and barriers to progress. Nevertheless it is planning the next stages in the change management process, which include exploring ways of delegating power further down the organisational hierarchies, establishing more self-managing teams, and, perhaps most challenging of all, creating a resource slack so it is possible for the organisation and its staff to develop and initiate change, not just react.

Social change was central to many of the initiatives set up (and mostly very quickly closed down again) through the Government's Community Development Programme (CDP) which was explored earlier in Chapter 1. Many issues raised through community initiatives, be they concerned with regeneration, health or young people, are beyond the role and remit of local people and local organisations to change, for example in relation to welfare benefit regulations and levels, or the ultimate levels of funding and resourcing available to local organisations such as health authorities and local authorities. Bodies such as the Association of Metropolitan Authorities (AMA); the NHS Confederation (previously known as the National

Table 11.1   Aims and methods in health promotion (from Ewles and Simnett 1992, p. 91)

AIM	APPROPRIATE METHOD
Health awareness goal Raising awareness, or consciousness, of health issues	Talks Group work Mass media Displays and exhibitions Campaigns
Improving knowledge Providing information	1-to-1 teaching Displays and exhibitions Written materials Mass media Campaigns Group teaching
Self-empowering Improving self-awareness, self-esteem, decision making	Group work Practising decision making Values clarification Social skills training Simulation, gaming and role play Assertiveness training Counselling
Changing attitudes and behaviour Changing the lifestyles of individuals	Group work Skills training Self-help groups 1-to-1 instruction Group or individual therapy Written material Advice
Social/environmental change Changing the physical or social environment	Positive action for under-served groups Lobbying Pressure groups Community development Community-based work Advocacy schemes Environmental measures Planning and policy making Organisational change Enforcement of laws and regulations

Association of Health Authorities and Trusts – NAHAT), as well as professional bodies and associations (e.g. Society of Health Education and Promotion Specialists – SHEPS) and networking/co-ordinating bodies (such as the Standing Conference for Community Development – SCCD) provide forums where issues that get raised at local levels by local communities or communities of interest can become the subject of national lobbying, and in the case of pressure groups, campaigning, particularly if similar issues are being raised in communities in other parts of the country.

In any particular community health initiative it may be that work is being undertaken in relation to a number of levels of change. A useful exploration of levels of change in relation to promoting health can be found in Ewles and Simnett's *Promoting Health: A Practical Guide* (1992) (see previous page). Clearly the methods and approaches used by health promoters vary depending on the level of change envisaged. For example, is change to take place at the level of the individual or wider community? There are many who argue that work to promote health and well-being and to prevent accidents and disease needs to work on a range of levels. Indeed, a CD approach to health grew out of the recognition that people's lifestyles cannot be seen in isolation from their social and economic environments.

Linking community development and organisation development

The history of community development (CD) in the UK has shown that much of the radical energy of the late 1960s and 1970s has now become institutionalised as CD becomes part of mainstream work. In community health work, for example, most of the early community health projects grew up from the voluntary sector in response to locally defined and perceived needs. Their position in the voluntary sector left them free to take on an outside 'lobbying' role, directly challenging the health and social welfare systems. In the 1980s and 1990s community development work has gained a place within existing NHS and social care systems, with many community health initiatives now directly funded by, and situated within, the statutory sector. As well as contradictions there are obviously clear practical advantages from this. Working 'within the system' requires some different skills and approaches, but can also have tactical advantages in terms of being able to influence change from within. Alinsky (1972) had discussed this issue in the 1960s when exploring community development work in the US:

As an organiser I start from where the world is, as it is, not as I would like it to be. That we accept the world as it is does not in any sense weaken our desire to change it into what we believe it should be – it is necessary to begin where the work is if we are going to change it to what we think it should be. That means working in the system. [p. xix]

Working 'within the system', that is, working with communities to bring about changes in the factors and services which effect their health and health care provision, requires the understanding of how organisations function, and how to bring about changes within them.

Organisation development (OD) is concerned with change, and in particular with the management of change; for this reason it is one of the most obviously relevant 'management' theories in relation to CDH work. However, another often-promoted feature of OD is that it should be 'top led' which immediately separates it from a community development approach to change (which is promoted as 'bottom up'). Apart from the polarised starting points for change, the actual techniques and features of OD and CD are often very similar. OD focuses on harnessing the human energy within an organisation by realising the full potential of the people within the organisation. It assists the effectiveness, capabilities and adaptability of the organisation by improving the processes by which people get things done and the relationships between people and groups within the organisation. If the word 'community' is substituted for organisation the statement above has a familiar ring to CD work.

It is possible to draw many parallels between OD and CD. This is helpful for two reasons. First it helps CD and CDH workers to recognise that the skills they have acquired from working directly with communities may also be useful in helping to bring about changes in systems and structure. Second, it can help managers realise that the participatory management approaches and skills that feature heavily on MBA courses and in popular management textbooks (e.g. Kanter 1985; Peters 1987) apply as much to their dealings with local communities and service users as they do to their own staff and organisational management roles. Some parallels between CD and OD are explored below:

- Both are deliberate strategies to manage, rather than merely respond to, change.
- Both see the process (i.e. how the work is carried out) as crucial in influencing the outcome(s).
- Both require a range of facilitative and catalytic skills.
- Both are crucially concerned with politics (with a small 'p') and power issues.

- Both place major emphasis on people's motivation to change, and on understanding and finding ways to overcome resistance to change.
- Both concentrate on maximising group and individual potential.
- Both regard change as inevitable, ongoing and dynamic.
- Group and leadership theories play a crucial role in analysis and practice.
- Involvement and participation of key stakeholders are important to both approaches.
- Both work on a number of different levels; i.e. individual, group, inter-group and whole organisation/strategic.

OD and CD also follow similar stages in terms of a structured and strategic approach to change:

- Gaining entry (to group, community, organisation, situation).
- Building up contacts and trust; clarifying the 'change agent' role.
- Identifying formal and informal groups, networks and structures.
- Working with others to identify the main problems, opportunities and areas of concern or common interest.
- Identifying what people want/need to change.
- Collectivising commitment and getting involvement in achieving the change(s).
- Clarifying openings and blocks (identifying 'friends' and 'enemies').
- Start to use tools, techniques and methods to bring about the desired changes.
- Evaluate.
- Continue the next stage of the process.

OD draws on both behavioural sciences and the specific business and environmental issues relating to an organisation. In practice, OD intervention takes place at a number of different levels. In theory these should be tackled consequentially, in practice there is often intervention happening at several different levels at the same time.
The levels are:

- Personal   e.g. inter-personal skills; clarifying individual roles and responsibilities.
- Group   e.g. problem solving; team/group development.
- Inter-group   e.g. relations between different parts of an organisation; conflict management.
- Structural/organisation   e.g. planning systems; communication structures.

These levels of working are also familiar to community health work. Again, in theory they evolve sequentially but in practice people are usually operating on all four levels at any one time. For example, the worker may make contact with individuals through a local well women's clinic, they may set up a self-help group, the group may link (inter-group level) to other women's health groups in the area to form a network or organise a collective event. The network may then link with the local health authority (structural level) to bring about change in relation to women's health (e.g. a new type of service, or changes to an existing service) (Smithies 1991, pp. 243–44).

Two publications by the Community Development Foundation explore the OD implications of work at community development levels. The first, *Organisational Development in the Community: Application, Tools and Discussion* (Batson and Smith 1995) is concerned with identifying practical use of OD approaches with a range of community groups. The second, *Gaining Ground: Support Pack for Community Groups* (May and Skinner 1995), explores OD for community groups and organisations (i.e. how they can be helped to develop as small-scale organisations in their own right).

Community Matters is a national voluntary organisation which works to support and network small community organisations, particularly those concerned with running community buildings such as community centres or social clubs. They too have recognised the need for OD skills and resources to support local community initiatives and activity. A national training and development programme, Community Matters Facilitation Training, has been established by them to help develop a national network of 'community consultants', i.e. people who can work with local community groups and organisations to help them manage change.

Tools for change

Whether change is at the level of individuals, community, organisation or wider society there are a range of tools and techniques which can be used to help people explore change management issues, from why change is necessary through to the best ways of moving change forward. The following examples give a flavour of some of the techniques which are around.

Force field analysis

This is an analytical tool that can be used very simply, or developed to a more sophisticated level. The most basic force field analysis relies on a grid as depicted.

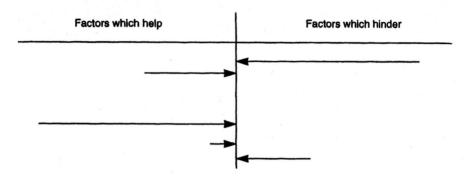

Figure 11.2   Force field analyis grid

The idea is to plot as an individual, or as part of a group exercise, factors which at present (or might in the future if the initiative is one that is planned rather than already underway) help or hinder a particular initiative or situation. Other terminology is sometimes used instead of helping and hindering, such as restraining and stimulating, for example.

The exercise can be made more sophisticated if arrows are used to indicate the 'strength' of each force (see diagram above). The longer the arrow, the greater the force. A further level of sophistication can be added by putting relevant sub-categories within the overall diagram (for example political, personal, skills, economics, etc.) and then logging the helping and hindering forces under each sub-heading.

Force field analysis can be useful in illustrating differing views between people, and in helping to pinpoint blocks or fears and concerns. However, its real use comes once the forces have all been logged. It is then important to look at how to move forward. This could be a matter of devising tactics to deal with the hindering or restraining forces, or to build up on the helping or stimulating forces, or both.

Strengths, weaknesses, opportunities and threats (SWOT)

'SWOT', as it is known, is a similar but perhaps slightly more sophisticated tool than Force Field Analysis. A grid is used (for example, a sheet of flip-chart paper, divided into four quarters as shown in Figure 11.3). Each of the four grids represents either strengths, weaknesses, opportunities or threats. As a general rule of thumb, strengths and weaknesses are current, opportunities and threats are based on future projections.

The exercise can be used with individuals or groups, and is a way of clarifying people's perspectives on either the whole or part of the organisation and group, or a particular project or work task. The exercise needs time

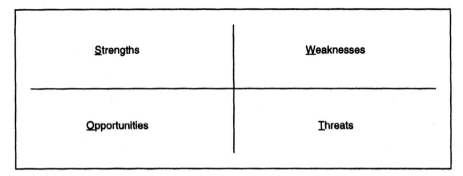

Figure 11.3 The SWOT grid

to follow through once people have listed their views under each of the SWOT headings. People may not always agree which heading something should go under; for instance, one person may see something as a strength, another as a weakness, so time is needed to explore different perspectives. Time is also needed to help people quantify the different things on their grid, e.g. there may be ten strengths and only five weakness, but one or two of the weaknesses may be so profound that they leave people feeling fairly negative despite all the strengths. People will also need time, and perhaps encouragement, to look at ways of dealing with weaknesses and threats, and at ways of turning opportunities into real practical action. They will also need to look at ways of building on their strengths and of using their strengths to help with the other three categories on the grid.

This could be used, for example, with a community health group to look at health services on their estate, or with a Primary Care Group to assess their approach to public involvement in purchasing.

Circles of influence

This technique (devised by Andrew Leigh, 1988) is helpful either in its own right or alongside tools such as SWOT and Force Field Analysis, as it can be used to help people further assess the weaknesses/threats and hinder categories. As with all these techniques it can be used with individuals or groups. The technique is basically concerned with problem solving (hence the link with the 'negatives' aspects of SWOT and Force Field). People are asked to identify all the issues they currently perceive as problems or difficulties. These then need to be brought together into one list if people have broken down into smaller groups for the initial stage, and any vague statements tightened up. They are then asked to say whether each problem is rated A, B or C, based on the grid in Figure 11.4 set out below.

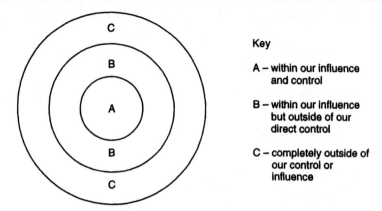

Key

A – within our influence and control

B – within our influence but outside of our direct control

C – completely outside of our control or influence

Figure 11.4   'Circles of influence' analysis

This stage may need lots of debate, but eventually people should agree which of their problems/difficulties are A, B or C. People will then need to think creatively about how to take immediate action to remedy the As; how best to exert influence on the Bs, and how to let go of the Cs, as they will simply be building up frustration and wasting time when very little can be achieved. However, it is also worth helping people to look at whether the boundaries around A, B and C can be shifted, before finalising the exercise and action plan.

This could be used with a community group to help people look at factors which affect their health; it could also be done within an organisation or team to help people who are feeling demoralised about starting or completing an initiative because they perceive it to be beset by problems.

Responsibility charting

This is best used when working with a team or group of people, particularly people who are working on complex issues or team/group projects that require lots of different tasks within the whole project. It can be especially useful at the end of a planning meeting or action planning day.

Again, a grid is used to map out the chart. The more visual this is (e.g. done on a piece of flip-chart paper) the more impact it is likely to have.

It is useful to list all the decisions or action points on a separate sheet of paper (this can be done during the day/meeting as things arise or by a group brainstorm just prior to carrying out this exercise). Each action point/task/decision needs to be then given a letter (A, B, C, etc.) and the sheet hung where everyone can see it. The reason for doing this is so that the responsibility chart does not get too complicated with words.

The chart itself should have everyone's name or initials along the top and all the action point references down the side (in Figure 11.5 below there are five people in the group and five action points).

People / Tasks	Amina	Akhtar	Jane	Mercy	Raymond
A	✔				
B		✔		⊘	
C		✔	⊘		✔
D					✔

Figure 11.5 Responsibility charting: an example

The idea is then to go through each task or action point and decide who is going to take things forward. A tick is put against the conjunction of the person and the task. For example, task A will be undertaken by Amina. Task B is to shared by Akhtar and Mercy. Task C shared by three of the group, and so forth. When more than one person is involved in following up action it is important to indicate which person will take the lead in getting the pair or group organised to take the task or action forward. This can be done, as indicated in the diagram above, by circling the appropriate person/task tick.

This exercise is useful for a number of reasons; it ensures that action on ideas and decisions is taken forward; it highlights who is volunteering and who is not; it can also highlight who has the power to act and who does not; it can highlight who is taking on too much responsibility (or holding on to power?). It can also provide a useful checklist to return to at a future meeting, and show how different tasks and roles contribute towards the achievement of a large scale and/or complex initiative.

This technique can be used, for example, by a community group planning a health day, or by an inter-sectoral Health For All partnership taking action after a planning workshop.

Commitment planning

This exercise (based on Beckhard and Harris 1987) involves identifying key players, who may be groups or individuals, in a given situation and trying to determine what their point of view or approach is likely to be. The object of the exercise is to determine tactics to move people from where they are perceived to be to where they need to be if they are to help the project or activity to be successful. A chart/grid is drawn up as below in Figure 11.6. This example depicts a local health needs assessment for a housing estate. The key people/groups who have been identified are listed on the left side of the grid. The health visitor is perceived to be neutral at the moment – maybe she has not yet been approached to get involved; she needs to actively support the initiative, perhaps because she has lots of contacts with parents with young children and the elderly living in the area. The people carrying out this exercise will need to work out how they think they can get her actively supporting the venture.

The GP is perceived to be against the needs assessment; she or he needs to be moved into a position where they are neutral and the work can carry on without direct opposition. The people carrying out the needs assessment may have decided it is unrealistic to expect the GP to be supportive, and will settle for 'neutralising' their opposition.

The Councillor may be actively supporting the needs assessment, but may need to take a bit more of a back-seat support role so as to give local residents the chance to get involved and have a say too.

The Residents' Association are clearly already supportive – they may think such an initiative is a good idea, but the needs assessment may need their active involvement in very practical ways as well, so they may need to be encouraged to become actively supportive, not just supportive in principle.

The chart can be used as a group planning tool, or to analyse blocks and barriers within an initiative.

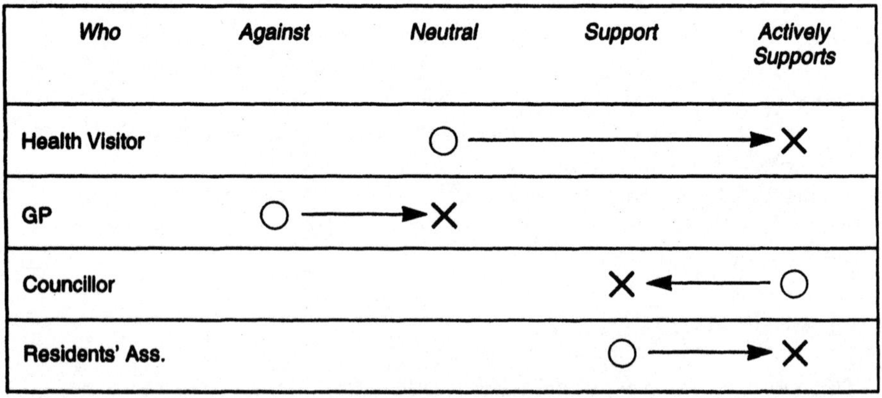

Who	Against	Neutral	Support	Actively Supports
Health Visitor		O ─────────────► X		
GP	O ───► X			
Councillor			X ◄──── O	
Residents' Ass.			O ───► X	

Figure 11.6   Commitment planning: an example

Iceberg analysis

This is another analytical tool (based on Plant 1987, pp. 128–9) which can be used for a range of purposes. For example, it can be helpful in determining why people hit problems and hitches; why people feel alienated or uncertain; who is holding on to power and control – and how and why. In this type of analysis, people indicate what they think goes on above the 'waterline' and what goes on below it.

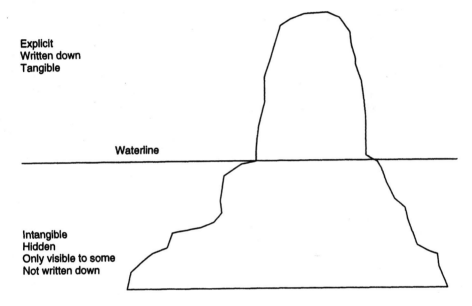

Figure 11.7   Iceberg analysis

Things that are above the waterline, i.e. the top of the iceberg, are clear for all to see; things below are not visible to everyone and are intangible. The sort of things that might be above the waterline are job descriptions or elected roles and responsibilities, lines of formal accountability, signatories to a joint-working/partnership agreement, stated aims and objectives. Below the waterline might be informal relationships and networks, alternative power and decision-making structures (e.g. in the pub after the meeting), expectations and assumptions.

As with real icebergs, although a watch can be appointed and a route plotted to sail around the visible and known part of the ice, the boat (i.e. individual/group/team/organisation) can be caught by the ice below the waterline, which may be much more rugged and uncertain. In many instances things below the waterline may not need to be. Much that goes on in teams, organisations and groups could be more formalised and made explicit, for example, expectations can be stated and logged. However, some things such as informal networks or assumptions are much harder to formalise and make explicit; there will always be some things that come below the waterline, but the line can be lowered so that more people can see more of the iceberg.

This exercise can illustrate differences between what is above or below the waterline for different people, for example, it may be useful when a group consisting of local people and/or service users and representatives of organisations has been brought together; it can also be used to look where things need to be firmed up or formalised and can help people see why they keep failing to make progress.

Examples of practical use include the management committee of a community centre which is failing to act in a co-ordinated way or a team of middle mangers in an organisation who are charged with a task (e.g. public involvement) but who fail to influence senior-level decision making. Another example is a partnership initiative which is just starting out and needs to address some informal as well as formal power-, resource- and information-sharing issues.

Stars

This is a tool[3] to help plot changes and developments, and also to help focus on achievements and priorities. It involves an individual or a team or group in plotting their work. A grid is used, as illustrated below.

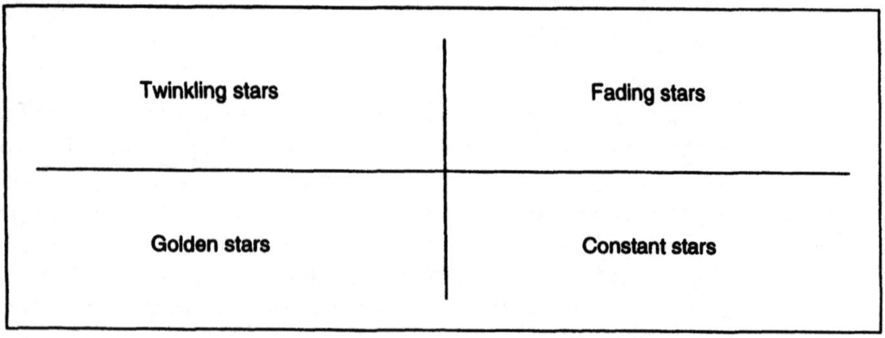

Twinkling stars	Fading stars
Golden stars	Constant stars

Figure 11.8   Stars analysis grid

Twinkling stars are new ideas or possibilities; fading stars are things that are on the way out for one reason or another; golden stars are the things that are specialities, things that the group or organisation excel at, and constant stars are the routine 'bread and butter', more mundane but nevertheless important tasks or roles that keep things ticking over.

As with all the other examples, people are asked to plot what issues go under which heading, and look at whether things need to move between headings. For example, does a twinkling star really need to become a fading star if nothing has come of some initial work? Does a constant star need working up to become a golden star?

This could be used as part of a range of evaluation tools for a community group or as a way of deciding what to highlight in a funding application. It could be used by a team or group in an organisation fighting for more resources or planning for the year ahead.

Diamond nines

This is a technique which can be used to help people set priorities. If a fair number of people are involved, the exercise can take quite a long time. The initial task is to identify all the areas of interest or possible need or demand. If this list comes to more than nine items then the group need to eliminate some issues, either though negotiation or debate, or if time is short or discussion has become stuck, through voting. The next step is to break people down into smaller groups (pairs is ideal). Each pair are asked to use the nine priorities to create a diamond shape. The diamond is a technique for getting people to see how different priorities might link together and also a way of avoiding simply listing issues from one to nine. Something that ends up being at the apex of the diamond may not be felt to be the most important issue overall, but may need actioning first if some of the other issues further down in the pattern are to be progressed.

Figure 11.9   The diamond nines analysis

The pairs will need to produce a diamond shape as above, each X representing one of the nine previously agreed priorities, and also to agree a rationale for why certain issues come higher or lower in the diamond.

Once this has been completed, groups need to be merged gradually; that is, after working in pairs, to be merged with another pair to be groups of four, again trying to agree upon a common diamond by sharing their layout and rationale and negotiating between them where movement is needed to reach a compromise. The fours should then be merged into eights, and so on. The eventual aim is to have one diamond that all present can agree on – or agreement about how competing priorities can be worked on if agreement is not forthcoming.

This exercise could be used by a community health group to help decide on priorities for topics to focus on, or within an organisation trying to decide which community groups to fund in the coming year.

Notes

1   French, W.L. and Bell, C.H. (1984), *Organisation Development*, Prentice Hall, 3rd edn. Quoted in Batson and Smith (1995), p. 37.
2   Presentation by Joan Durose, Combined Health Care Trust, to the CD/OD Network, Sheffield, 1996.
3   Based on a presentation by J. McAuley to students at the Sheffield Business School in February 1991.

Part III

Taking forward community involvement in health

This section contains chapters which explore what needs to change in organisations, in professional training and skills and in communities, if the potential of community involvement in health is to be fully realised. Checklists for action accompany these suggestions. This section also lists and describes some of the existing resources, contacts and agencies which can support this action.

Parts I and II describe the support that exists for community involvement in health, from central government, within organisations and within communities, and practical models that have been developed and used. However, the gains that have been made because of this support are patchy, varying between different parts of the country, different organisations and different communities. They are in danger of being lost and not built upon unless people at all levels of society continue to press for the necessary changes. This part of the book, by concentrating on changes designed to help individuals, organisations and communities shift from an ad hoc, one-off approach to community involvement, to a strategic and all-encompassing approach, aims to meet this gap.

12 A critical path to involvement

Summary

This chapter outlines a number of steps which organisations need to take to build a strategic approach to community involvement in health. The chapter begins with describing three sets of activities for all organisations concerned with community involvement. It is followed by a summary of the critical path to involvement and a description of each step in detail, with an example of how each one has been used in practice. It then considers some of the training and organisation development implications for organisations who wish to take forward this approach.

This critical path to involvement was originally developed by ourselves during research carried out for the then NHS Management Executive in 1993. This was research into the implications of 'responding to local voices' for purchasing organisations (Labyrinth 1993b). It was, therefore, developed with health authorities (as health purchasers and commissioners) in mind. It has been worked on and used since and with local adaptations, and can be used as a guide for all organisations wishing to pursue a strategic approach to community involvement in health.

Three sets of activities

Integral to any framework for community involvement in health is a threefold focus:

- Activities designed to reach out to consumers, patients, public and communities to find out their needs and views for ways forward.
- Activities designed to look within the organisation at the processes which need to change to accommodate those views.
- Activities designed to create an interface between the two so that a realistic, ongoing partnership is achieved.

Organisational stepping stones

The following directives constitute the 'stepping stones' of the critical path to involvement:

- *Audit current state of play* Map what is already going on in terms of community involvement in health in your organisation, and also in other local organisations including the voluntary sector.
- *Establish a clear, locally-based rationale* Why does your organisation want community involvement? How will you use the information and contacts that come out of such processes? Is everyone in the organisation in agreement, and clear about the implications; that is, is there corporate ownership?
- *Be clear about your relationship to stakeholders* Who else has an interest/stake in community involvement in health? Who else might be affected by the findings and outcomes of such work? Can you get them involved in the work from an early stage as partners in the initiative?
- *Clarify the degree of involvement you are aiming for* Be clear about the use of language, for example do you call something 'involvement' when really you are talking about 'consultation'? Be clear how much of a role the community will be able to play in influencing decisions.
- *Reach out to the community* Develop contacts, decide on methods and approaches to get involvement and take forward initiatives jointly with communities.
- *Look within the organisation* Are the structures, systems and skills within the organisation ones that support and enable community involvement? Are there mechanisms in place to ensure that needs that emerge can be actioned?
- *Develop the community/organisational interface* Are there formal mechanisms to ensure ongoing links to a community after a relationship has been established; to ensure ongoing feedback on progress; to continue a dialogue about new and changing needs; and so on? This interface

could be, for example, a community health forum, or a locality planning mechanism.

- *Organise the work* Who is going to take the lead on community involvement – one person? a small team? Are they at a senior enough position in the organisation to make sure that change happens? Have they got credibility with both the communities and staff and managers in the organisation?

These steps do not necessarily need to be taken in the order that they are described. It is more important that they are seen as a set of 'stepping stones' which, taken together, represent a critical path to involvement. It is also important that following the path is not seen as a one-off exercise. Each step will need revisiting at regular intervals, in part to monitor progress, but mainly to highlight new needs or gaps that will appear in the transition from seeing local people as 'recipients' of health services and health care, to their transformation as active 'participants' in the shaping and planning of those services. The transformation mentioned here is mainly concerned with changes that organisations need to make, internally as well as externally, although it also refers to the change in the way that local people see their own role in this process. The critical path will need revisiting because community involvement in health, along the lines envisioned in this book, is a developmental process. As organisations begin to open up, encourage local views and work in partnership with local people, so the views, attitudes and visions of all those involved in this process will develop. Thus the 'path to involvement' will be extended and new issues will emerge that will need to be addressed along the way.

The stepping stones in detail

Audit the current state of play

- What community groups and voluntary organisations with a broad health remit already exist in your area? Remember to distinguish between the two; Chapter 5 will help here.
- What mechanisms already exist within your organisation for including the community in your working groups and decision-making structures? Do you know of any within other relevant organisations?
- What resources exist within your organisation to support or develop community-based health initiatives? This might be in the form of

grants, worker time, or information and publicity. Do you know of any such resources within other relevant organisations?

Box 12.1   Review by Newcastle and North Tyneside Health Authority

The 1996/7 Corporate Contract developed by Newcastle and North Tyneside Health Authority states that the authority will 'review and evaluate present methods of public involvement, mapping out current position and identifying areas for improvement by May 1996 ...' This evaluation will help to look at what has been achieved and what needs to happen next to take public involvement forward in the District.

Establish a clear, locally-based rationale

- Why does your organisation want community involvement in health?
- What is your desired outcome, main concerns and focus? Are these reflected within the mission statement, aims and objectives of your organisation?
- How will you ensure that everyone in the organisation is in agreement and clear about the implications of your approach?
- Why do you think the local population will want to get involved with your organisation and its aims?
- How will you use the information and contacts that come out of the community involvement process?

Table 12.1   Community roles within an organisational health strategy

Advocacy	*Service provision*	*Gatekeepers*
On behalf of a specific group or specific health issues	Via grants, service contract with purchasers, subcontracts via providers, or independent resourcing	To wider general public

Needs assessment	*Empowerment*	*Partnership*
Through participatory methods	Through confidence-building, skills development, validation	Input into planning and development

- Using the model in Table 12.1 as a guide, what roles would you like community groups and voluntary organisations to play? What roles do you thing they will consider appropriate for themselves? How can you establish a dialogue with them about this?

Box 12.2   Bradford Health's Community Development Strategy

Bradford Health have adopted a Community Development Strategy for the Authority, which has been sanctioned at board level. The process of developing the strategy took about six months and was participatory, involving other key agencies, local community health projects and workers. The strategy lists six clear reasons, or rationale, for developing the work on community involvement:

- To move from the current position to a planned approach to community development.
- To prioritise a way of working within the eight 'Health of Bradford' target areas where disadvantage is a barrier to health.
- To recommend organisational changes that might need to take place to maximise the CD approach.
- To use as an educational tool for commissioners needing an understanding of CD and the organisational support required for its success.
- To produce a strategic plan that has had input from staff across the agencies who have expertise in CD.
- To contribute to the 'Inequalities in Health' project by proposing a practical way forward to address inequalities in health, and suggesting an investment plan designed to address inequalities in health.

Be clear about your relationship to stakeholders

- Who else in your area has an interest/stake in community involvement in health?
- What groups and organisations might be affected by the outcomes of your work to promote community involvement in health?
- How can you involve key stakeholders in your local 'healthy alliance' and how can you ensure that community involvement is a key aspect of this alliance?
- How can you encourage key stakeholders to build community involvement within their own organisation or group, e.g. through advice,

joint training, contract specifications, jointly organised community awareness-raising events?

The model below shows some key stakeholders from the perspective of health purchasing organisations. It can be adapted for use by other organisations and groups.

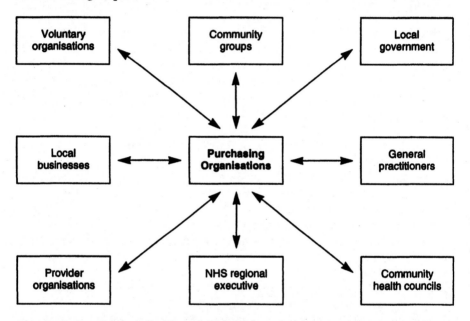

Figure 12.1   Key stakeholders for health purchasing organisations considering community involvement

---

Box 12.3   Healthy Alliances within North Staffordshire

North Staffordshire Health Authority shares its geographical area with three local authorities and part of a county council. In order to progress work in relation to partnership initiatives, health inequalities and community development, it has established three 'Healthy Alliance Partnerships', one within each of the three local authority areas. Each partnership has its own full-time worker attached, managed by the Health Authority, and each is chaired by a senior member of the Health Authority management team. The three Healthy Alliance workers are all involved directly with community development work as well as strategic level initiatives.

Clarify the degree of involvement you are aiming for

Using the 'ladder of participation' and other models described in Chapter 5 (Figure 5.1) as a guide:

● What degree of community involvement in health are you looking for in the long term for your organisation?
● What degree of community involvement can you realistically make a start with? This will probably vary with different population or user groups.
● Be clear and honest with local people about where your boundaries lie for community involvement and how much of a role the community will be able to play in influencing decisions. Be clear about language and do not talk about 'participation' when you really mean 'consultation'.
● Consider what further steps you will make to move closer to the degree of involvement you are looking for in the long term.

Box 12.4 Participatory health needs assessment in North Yorkshire

North Yorkshire Health Authority commissioned and carried out a participatory health needs assessment within one of its more deprived localities. This has been combined with organisation development work to explore with the communities involved, as well as partner agencies, the degree of involvement and participation they would like at area-based levels, and how this can be achieved. This led to the establishment of a community health forum with full involvement of key agencies and community representatives, with clear boundaries for participation and decision making.

Reach out to the community

The models, concepts and case studies in Part II will help you tackle these questions:

● Who makes up your local communities and what do you already know about their health needs? This will include considering demographic data, indices of deprivation, prior knowledge and so on.
● What communities or groups are your priorities in terms of seeking their involvement? This might be particular localities, population groups or user groups.

- How can you ensure that the needs of individuals and groups who have not traditionally been involved and/or heard, are specifically sought?
- What does your audit tell you about your current access to them?
- What participatory methods will you use to access them?
- How will you feed back to the community the results of their involvement?
- How else can you illustrate your commitment to building community involvement in health, to the local community?

There are examples of effective methods that can be used to 'reach out' to a range of different communities in Chapter 9 on 'participatory needs assessment'.

Look within the organisation

The following questions are mainly concerned with organisation development:

- Are the structures, systems and skills within the organisation ones that support and enable community involvement? How far is this the case within other organisations which form 'healthy alliances' with yourselves?
- Are there mechanisms in place that ensure that community needs that emerge can be actioned?
- What support is available within the organisation to help you build the systems, structures and skills required for community involvement? This support includes resources for training and organisation development, as well as the commitment of key individuals and groups within the organisation. Can you draw on support in these areas from other organisations you are in alliance with?
- What approaches do you want to adopt to build the appropriate structures, systems and skills?

Develop the community/organisational interface

- What current formal mechanisms exist for ongoing dialogue and feedback with the community?
- Are these mechanisms 'one-off' (e.g. public meetings) or developmental (e.g. community health forum, locality planning mechanism)?
- How can you make them developmental so that community involvement becomes a partnership activity?
- In what ways can you resource the community/voluntary sector in-

frastructure so that the community is enabled to develop the capacity to act as partners with yourselves?

● In what ways can you encourage other organisations to become part of a community/organisation interface, for example, through including community involvement requirements within contract specifications for providers?

Box 12.5   Linking organisation development to community involvement

Combined Health Care NHS Trust, which is based in North Staffordshire, has developed a coherent strategy to look at the organisation development implications of community involvement work. It is co-ordinated by the Director of Learning and Change for the Trust. The framework for staff development has three key areas, each of which is broken down into a number of competencies. They are: understanding our role in the community, managing the boundaries, and ensuring continuous improvement. They have an action plan for putting the strategy into practice.

Redbridge and Waltham Forest Health Authority carried out a review of its initiatives in relation to community involvement and what had changed as a result. Although a lot was going on, internal communication and decision-making structures were identified as blocks to progressing work to effect real changes in policy, contracts and priorities in relation to community involvement. They responded by carrying out an internal organisation development review and then developing a clear organisational framework for community involvement.

Box 12.6   Training consultation facilitators

Sheffield Health is a partner in Healthy Sheffield, together with other agencies. It played a key role in the major consultation exercise carried out by Healthy Sheffield, which sought the involvement of a wide range of communities, groups and organisations in the development of the city's health plan, 'Our City Our Health'. Thirty people from all sectors were trained as core trainers, and in turn trained 150 facilitators from all sectors to facilitate the involvement process. Their role was to enable discussions across the city about the key health issues facing local people and what should be done about them. This massive exercise led to the development and support of a number of mechanisms to ensure ongoing community involvement in health decisions – the 'interface'.

Organisation of the work

● Who within your organisation 'will take a lead on community involvement work – an individual or a team? Are they at a senior enough position within the organisation to ensure that change happens? Have they got credibility with both the community, and staff and managers within the organisation, or how will they build it?

● How will this work be reported to and discussed with the highest levels of the organisation, to maintain their commitment and ownership?

● Who will ensure that this work is co-ordinated, both within your organisation and within your 'healthy alliance' structure?

● What resources can you identify within the organisation that can help you carry out this work?

● What resources can be identified within your partner bodies such as local authorities and voluntary organisations that can help to carry out this work?

Box 12.7   Organising community involvement work

Public involvement work in Buckinghamshire Health Authority was led by the Director of Communications. She built up an integrated communications strategy and structure that allowed all parts of the Authority to set up and maintain direct two-way communications with the general public, service users and voluntary organisations as well as other key partner agencies. Acute services provided an initial focus for community participation work, along with the three Health For All initiatives in the county.

Key messages for health purchasers

This section describes some of the key messages for health purchasers who wish to promote and take forward community involvement in health and in their own and allied organisations. These messages derive from the experience of a wide range of people working within health organisations on community involvement. They are taken from the Labyrinth research for the NHS Management Executive mentioned earlier (Labyrinth 1993b, pp. 3–4), and from a more recent review of community participation in health purchasing within England (Labyrinth 1996b, p. 6). They were reinforced by participants from health authorities, NHS trusts, community health councils, local authorities and voluntary organisations at a recent national workshop held in Manchester (Labyrinth 1993b, p. 2).

- Community involvement needs to be a top priority for purchasing organisations in order to develop the commitment and action necessary for the large-scale change required.
- Top management and Board-level commitment is needed, providing a lead to the organisation as a whole about the importance of community involvement. Commitment needs to be extended to all levels.
- Commitment to community involvement in health requires a major shift, 'transformational' rather than 'transitional', in the way health authorities are used to doing things, in their organisational systems, structures and cultures.
- Training and organisation development are crucial in taking forward community involvement in a way that creates real change.
- Community involvement implies ongoing participation of local communities rather than one-off consultation.
- Realistic timescales and a long-term plan are needed, that allows trust and infrastructures to be built up, and time for attitudes, skills and knowledge to develop and change.
- Different skills and approaches will be necessary for different types of community involvement and with different communities.
- Organisations need to develop a comprehensive, resourced and managed strategy for community involvement, with a clearly designated lead post and dedicated staff time to develop initiatives and projects. At the same time this work needs to be integrated at all organisational levels.
- Healthy alliances are a major part of a community involvement strategy, as the activities of a range of organisations impinge on people's health and well-being.
- It is important to achieve some small-scale successes which can be transformed into visible action as a response to community views and ideas, to maintain their involvement.
- Resources and support are necessary to enable community groups to develop their experience and skills in working with the health service and other agencies.
- It is important to evaluate different initiatives and to monitor achievements and blocks.

Training and organisation development

In the broad sense, taking a strategic approach to community involvement in health is an integral part of organisation development. However, this section focuses more specifically on the training and organisation work necessary to help build that strategy and make it effective.

A corporate approach to training and organisation development implies:

- Staff development to build a committed, creative and collective work force that is effective but remains flexible and open.
- Training as part of a change-management strategy to build the required skills, knowledge and attitudes.
- Organisation development to enable the organisation to change its values, culture, behaviour and structure to respond effectively to community involvement.
- Acknowledging the connection between these approaches. Training can be one part of carrying out organisation development, whilst particular training courses will throw up wider organisation development implications that need addressing.

A useful and practical way in to dealing with these issues is the identification of training needs. We then consider different methods which can be used for training and organisation development, to meet the identified needs, and how these activities might be resourced.

Identifying training needs

Table 12.2 is a guide to some of the training needs regarding community involvement which might be identified for key workers with key responsibility for community involvement within organisations, staff and members within the organisation as a whole, and for the voluntary and community sectors. They are a guide only and each local situation will throw up a number of other needs.

Different methods for training and organisation development

The following sections are not an exhaustive list and can be used in a 'mix and match' sort of way, depending on local situations and local needs. All these methods are suitable for use within and between organisations, at different levels, and with community groups. Clearly the way they are introduced and used will vary with the participant group.

Box 12.8   Training community representatives

Salford and Trafford Health Authority, with outside help, carried out a training needs analysis of community representatives from different ethnic minority communities in their Old Trafford locality. Following this, a training programme was developed and carried out, designed to build the skills, knowledge and confidence of community representatives. As a result they were enabled to carry out health needs assessments within their own communities which were fed into the authority's strategic planning structures. There were twelve training sessions, focusing on:

- How the NHS works.
- Health and socio-economic profile of the Old Trafford area.
- Recruitment and selection.
- The role of a community representative.
- Mental health.
- Rights and complaints.
- Interesting practice from elsewhere.
- Skills for community representatives.
- Community care.
- Focus groups and undertaking research in our own communities.
- Funding and finance.
- Bringing it all together.

Cascade training

This can be used both as a specific training tool, for instance to develop specific skills throughout the organisation as a whole, or as part of an organisation development approach aimed at getting collective involvement and ownership of certain issues and attitudes.

Basically cascade training works on a 'training the trainers' basis, starting with a group of people who are trained to take forward work with colleagues or other groups of people. It is an effective way of taking large numbers of people through a common process, and also extends understanding, ownership and commitment.

Table 12.2   A guide to identifying training needs

Key workers with lead responsibility	Staff and members of the whole organisation	Voluntary and community sectors
Knowledge: • Of voluntary sector • Of local area • Of NHS structures and policies, nationally and locally • Of structures of and contacts with other key organisations • Community involvement theory	**Knowledge:** • Of what is already going on re: community involvement in NHS and other sectors • Of local voluntary sector • Audit of organisation development needs • Audit of organisational training needs	**Knowledge:** • How purchasing works, planning cycle, role and remit of purchasing and other organisations • How to gain access to planning mechanisms, resources, grants • Of the range of the local community and voluntary sector and key contacts
Skills: • Managing change • Managing conflict negotiation • Communication • Understanding and achieving cultural change • Problem-solving tools and techniques • Public relations, presentation, media • Time/stress management, prioritisation • Listening • Research • Team building • Project management • Analytical • Community involvement tools and techniques	**Skills:** • Visioning for the future • Changing the organisational culture • Changing issues into policy • Participatory management • Internal communication • Team building • Public relations • Managing change • Alliance building • Conflict management • Feedback techniques (to local people)	**Skills:** • Assertiveness • Influencing decision making and change • Presentation • Communication • Marketing • Financial and budgeting • Survey/interviewing • Identifying training needs • Group work/advocacy
Attitudes: • Cultural awareness (different communities) • Social awareness (different needs) • Equal opportunities	**Attitudes:** • Commitment across whole organisation • Ownership across whole organisation • Opening up the organisation to wider influence • Equal opportunities • Corporate identity • Encouragement and promotion of innovation • Flexible working practices	**Attitudes:** • Awareness of what being representative means • Equal opportunities • Enthusiasm and staying power

Facilitated workshops

Giving people the chance to take time out, as groups, teams and individuals, creates the opportunity to free up thinking from day-to-day pressures and deadlines. It allows complex situations to be shared and analysed, and joint plans for action to be developed. A good facilitator is essential.

Team development

This helps existing teams to work well together. It is also an important part of building a new team, whether it is a team internal to one organisation, or one with members drawn from a range of organisations and sectors. Team development can help to clarify roles and responsibilities within a group, develop an organised and committed way of working, and build a shared vision and action plans to meet the vision. It is especially important in helping inter-sectoral groups form and organise.

Using the IPR scheme

Many organisations have adopted an 'Independent Performance Review' scheme for their staff. Assessing training needs is an important function of the scheme. Good-quality reviewing and follow-up support should help people assess their learning, review next steps and consider longer change management implications. When the IPR scheme works effectively, managers can use it to ensure that corporate objectives, such as community involvement, are integrated into individual and team objectives, and to build an overview of organisation development and training implications for their staff as a whole.

Inter-sectoral working groups

Sometimes such groups are organised so that the experiences of different members are shared as a formal part of the agenda of the group's meeting. This facilitates learning from the experience of others and can help the group as a whole move forward. However, such sharing needs to be carefully structured and facilitated so that lessons can be pulled out and action points noted.

Using local people and service users as trainers

This is a developing area and presents many challenges, including putting the user or local person in the 'professional' role of trainer, and the professionals in the role of participants.

Individual consultancy for key people

There may be insufficient skills and knowledge within the organisation to provide relevant support for staff with a community involvement brief. Non-managerial supervision can be a useful way of bridging that gap.

Organisational consultancy

Bringing in outside consultants can be a way of helping an organisation move forward with a community involvement brief. This can be for one-off sessions such as facilitating a workshop, or for longer-term consultancy work. This can include organisational reviews, developing a strategy, commitment planning or helping an organisation manage a complex change in the culture, structures and mechanisms required for community involvement.

Resources for training and organisation development

These will be necessary. Some organisations set aside a budget for their own internal training and organisation development needs; some of this can be set aside for work which enables community involvement. Equally, there will need to be resources set aside for a training fund for the voluntary and community sector so that they are enabled to participate actively and strategically in joint activities. It is also useful if training, workshops and consultancy can be organised on an intersectoral basis, so that visions, as well as skills, knowledge and ideas, can be shared. In this case the funding of such work can also be shared, which in turn helps to develop a message of co-operation.

13 Five elements of a community involvement in health strategy

Summary

This chapter focuses on a model which has been developed by the authors of this book, and used with many health authorities and boards and with multi-agency initiatives in terms of planning, mapping and evaluating community development and health work strategically. A case study of the way this model has been used in practice is also included.

Outline of the model

Labyrinth Training and Consultancy have developed a model for community development and health work which is entitled 'Five Essential Elements of a Community Involvement Strategy'. It has developed out of many years of working with organisations and communities to take forward meaningful community involvement. The model, Figure 13.1, is based on five inter-related elements.

Applying the model

The model has been used in both the form shown and in adapted forms by a wide range of organisations and initiatives, for example as the basis for a local area community development and health strategy in Kirkby in Knowsley (Labyrinth 1994a). It was also used as the basis for designing an

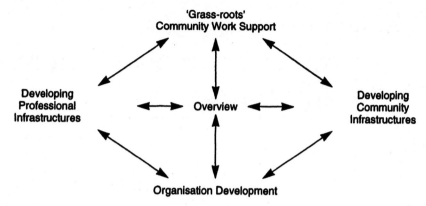

Figure 13.1   Five essential elements of a community involvement strategy

evaluation framework for the twenty or so initiatives across Wales which come together under Health Promotion Wales' 'Communities for Better Health' network (Community Development Foundation and Labyrinth 1996); as a model for undertaking an evaluation of a ten-year community development initiative based in a community health trust in Hackney, London (Labyrinth 1996c), and as the basis for a successful Single Regeneration Budget bid in Chesterton, North Staffordshire (Labyrinth 1995f). At the end of this chapter, the Kirkby work will be used as a case study to show how the model was applied to a real piece of work.

The model is based on the assumption that a strategic approach is needed to community involvement if it is going to effect real change. It suggests that work needs to happen at all five levels, and although the same individuals may not be involved at all five levels, all the work needs to be co-ordinated and linked into an overview.

The five elements in detail

Community work support

This involves development work in the community to enable individuals, especially from 'usually excluded' communities, to get together and organise around issues that they define as important to them. This will result in them setting up their own groups, pressing for participation in services, or influencing district/city policies.

Community infrastructure

This develops from community work and involves helping community and user groups and development workers to network with each other, to enable them to learn from each other and exchange information and support, so that they can move forward collectively. It helps them to learn from each other's successes and mistakes so that they do not have to 'reinvent the wheel'. It means that views from a number of different groups and communities can be gathered together.

Professional infrastructure

The aim of this element is to ensure that departments, organisations, individual managers and service delivery staff are networked with each other and are able at all levels to feed in information and ideas and thus be fully involved in developing inter-sectoral and inter-departmental policies and · services. It is important that they meet to exchange information and ideas, and clarify and develop roles and skills that encourage participation, and in so doing, support 'grass-roots' community work activity.

Organisation development

Organisation development aims to improve the effectiveness of the organisation through encouraging participation and responding to the needs and ideas from local communities and users of services. It involves creating an organisational environment which is open, has a long-term outlook, and which develops a strategy for effective change management in a participatory way. It means addressing issues of power, organisational culture and putting in place systems and structures that are publicly accountable and able to respond to new information, priorities and needs.

Overview

The elements described above are interdependent. Different people working at different levels within organisations, and from different sectors, will be primarily involved with different elements. Usually, for instance, community-based work is seen as completely separate from organisation development. They are undertaken by different workers, from different backgrounds within different strategic frameworks. If community involvement is to be taken seriously, it is important to link community work with the need for organisational change, so that local ideas and needs can affect wider policy, planning and practice. Therefore an overview is required which ensures coherence. It is important for co-ordination, but also to ensure that a strategic direction is followed.

What the model means in practice

Listed below are some examples of how to put the five basic elements of the strategic approach to involving local people into practice. These ideas are based on current practice within different organisations. It is important that work is carried out on each of the five elements if real change is to be achieved.

Without community work support to 'usually excluded' communities, the only groups whose voices would be heard within organisations would be the more articulate, vocal, organised ones. On the other hand, without organisation development the needs of communities, articulated through community work organising and community infrastructure networking, will find difficulty in finding an audience, and still less a chance of achieving changes in plans, policies, resource allocation and services. If professionals are excluded then not only is a useful potential resource overlooked, but also possible blocks and opposition may arise. If there is no co-ordination and overview then many people and projects may be working away without combining to achieve common overall goals and changes.

The ideas are looked at both from the point of view of an organisation-wide strategic approach (for example a health authority/local authority/City Challenge) and from the perspective of a locally based community development project, to illustrate both the need to be strategic at all levels of community involvement work, whether working with just one local community or with just one community project, or across a whole town or district with a wide range of community initiatives and inter-sectoral partnership working. Figure 13.2 below also indicates how work at these two levels overlaps.

'Grass-roots' community work support

The strategic approach at organisational level involves:

- Funding community/community health/user development workers.
- Setting up a small grants fund to enable community activity.
- Payment of expenses to enable participation e.g. child care, signers, transport.

Strategic approach at local community
development project level

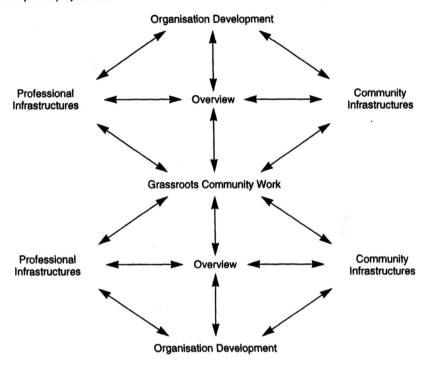

Figure 13.2 The five elements: project and organisational perspectives

- Help 'in kind' such as allowing free use of buildings for community meetings and events.

The strategic approach at local Community Development Project level includes:

- Meeting local people and identifying gaps and priorities in their local community.
- Setting up community groups and initiatives based on needs and interests.
- Supporting campaigns.
- Helping with funding applications.

Community infrastructure

The strategic approach at organisational level includes:

- Supporting city/district-wide forums such as Black Health Forum, Federation of Community Organisations, Network of Tenants Associations.
- Supporting accessible centralised information resources.
- Funding/offering district/city-wide training opportunities.

The strategic approach at local Community Development Project level includes:

- Organising community forums.
- Organising community-wide events such as festivals, play schemes.
- Getting a community news sheet off the ground.
- Undertaking a community profile.

Professional infrastructure

The strategic approach at organisational level includes:

- Offering community work skills training for community-based staff.
- Allowing time in work loads, job descriptions for group work and supporting community activity.
- Giving clear guidance on, and openings for, staff to feed in their perceptions of community needs and issues arising in local areas.
- Allowing time in job specs for professionals to attend inter-agency/multi-disciplinary forums.

The strategic approach at local Community Development Project level includes:

- Setting up a local workers' forum.
- Attending staff/team meetings of locally based organisations (e.g. social services, schools, health centre).
- Offering training/joint working opportunities to local professionals.
- Supply all local professionals with a community profile and encourage them to pass on information and contacts to their local 'clients'/service users.

Organisation development

The strategic approach at organisational level includes:

- Clarifying and establishing organisational policy and aims for community involvement.
- Developing an equal opportunities statement of intent, policy, practice guidelines and targets.
- Setting community involvement objectives and targets for each part of the organisation.
- Looking at ways of creating an organisational culture that encourages and enables participation and empowerment.
- Offer managers training in community involvement and managing change.
- Exploring organisation structures and systems to look at blocks in turning needs into action/policy change.

The strategic approach at local Community Development Project level includes:

- Supporting local people to get involved in the planning and management of the project.
- Making the project base as accessible as possible so people call in with ideas and requests for support.
- Holding open meetings to share what the project has been doing and invite ideas for what the project should be doing next.

Overview

The strategic approach at organisational level includes:

- Setting clear aims for the strategy.
- Establishing a Co-ordinating Group to take forward the community involvement strategy.
- Sharing the strategic development and thinking with other agencies.
- Appointing a worker at middle/senior management level to co-ordinate the strategy.
- Holding a city/district-wide annual event/conference to ensure a dialogue between strategic planners and grassroots workers and activists.
- Reviewing and monitoring the effectiveness of the strategic approach.

The strategic approach at local Community Development Project level includes:

● Involving people in monitoring and evaluation.
● Ensuring proper support and supervision for project workers.
● Developing and reviewing regular objectives and action plans for each piece of work and the project as a whole.

Using this model in your own work

This model has often been used on training courses or during planning and review workshops to help participants map where the emphasis is for their own work and where there is room for development, and to look at who else needs to be involved if an overall strategic approach is to be achieved. It has proved to be helpful when looking at the ways a number of organisations working together can contribute to an overall strategic approach, for example in relation to a Healthy City/ Health For All type initiative, where agencies are working together to take forward community participation in terms of both their practice and principles.

The model also adapts to other participation initiatives. For example, it has been used to help develop a framework for a user and carer participation strategy in Barnsley, South Yorkshire (Labyrinth 1995d). People involved in the development of advocacy services have also usefully adapted it to fit their work.

A model is only useful if it helps people focus on their practice, analyse strengths and gaps, and decide on ways forward to meet those gaps. Readers may wish to have a go themselves at using the model as an analytical and planning tool for their own work, either individually or with other people from communities, projects, their own organisations or multi-agency forums.

Case Study: The 'Five Elements' approach to needs assessment, and a community development and health strategy for Kirkby

Knowsley Council (which houses the Healthy Knowsley initiative), St Helen's and Knowsley Health Authority and the St Helen's and Knowsley Community Health NHS Trust came together, with ourselves as outside consultants, to undertake a health needs assessment in Kirkby. Kirkby is an area which has its own distinct boundaries, but which also has a number of smaller specific communities within it. It has a strong community spirit, and there is a history of community development and community activism. However, it is also an area of high deprivation and its population experiences poor health compared to the rest of the district (and in relation to national averages).

The needs assessment process was undertaken over the course of about four months, and included mapping current activity, and exploring needs through focus group discussions with the varied mix of community groups and residents. The main aim of the health needs assessment exercise was to identify ways in which health might be improved in the area, and in particular to look at ways of linking community participation more directly into the health purchasing function. To this end a community involvement in health strategy was produced, which included recommendations for action.

The model that has been described in the earlier part of this chapter was used, both as a way of mapping current activity and gaps, and also as a structure for presenting the recommendations. When this work was undertaken (in 1993/4) the model had only four elements; the 'overview' element was added as a result of both undertaking the needs assessment, and following work to get the recommendations taken forward by both single agencies, and in terms of multi-agency working. A small multi-agency group oversaw all the work from the initiation of the needs assessment through to getting the recommendations actioned. The group was made up of three local authority representatives (Healthy Knowsley, Social Services and Community Development); four health authority representatives (research and information, health gain and locality purchasing); one trust representative (health promotion), and the two Labyrinth consultants. The group continued to meet for some time after our consultancy work was completed. This group clearly undertook the 'overview' function, and it became obvious that without a group of people (or even a key individual) to hold things together, and to make connections and links between the other four elements of the model, then very little would have happened once the action stage was reached. Thus the model progressed to having five key elements.

The recommendations for action were all based on the findings from the needs assessment process. They are summarised below to give a feel of how the model was used in practice. The recommendations were organised under the five key elements:

1 Action to develop the grass roots.

   ● Establishment of a small grants fund.

- Review of charging policy within local community centres to enable new and/or unfunded groups to meet there.
- Exploration of ways of purchasing organisations contracting with local voluntary organisations in Kirkby to undertake community development and health work.
- Building in community development work to the contract between the health authority and the community trust.

2 Action to develop the community infrastructure.

- Community development newsletter to ensure more effective publicising of events and activities, and better sharing of information and opportunities.
- Training for community groups in relation to community development skills, and ideas for promoting health and organising to get action around health concerns and services.

3 Action to develop the professional infrastructure.

- Breaking down locality planning for Kirkby to smaller sub-areas so areas of particular need and deprivation are not lost within the whole.
- Training and development work with staff of key local agencies to promote a wider understanding of, and support for, community development ways of working.

4 Action to develop the organisational level.

- Review of the role of community nurses based in the area to look at the potential for increased time and resources being channelled into community development work.
- Review of the role of local authority services providers based in the area to look at the potential for increased time and resources being channelled into community development work.
- More co-ordinated policy lead within the local authority to ensure the Council as a whole is 'neighbourhood friendly'.
- More co-ordination at senior management levels of the key agencies in relation to jointly commissioning services and initiatives from main stream (not just joint finance resources).
- Top-level lead to empower staff of key agencies to work in ways that are about involving local residents and community groups as part of their day-to-day approach to working in Kirkby.

5 Action to develop and overview.

- Appointment of a Community Development and Health Manager for Kirkby to co-ordinate work across the area.

- Establishment of a Community Health Forum.
- Plan ways of meeting gaps identified in the needs assessment in relation to particular groups (e.g. young people's health, support work with carers).
- Development of a 'locality centre' ('one-stop shop'-type of initiative) for Kirkby, with full community involvement in the design, location and services offered.

Three years on almost all of these action points have been taken forward, and work in relation to community development and health in Kirkby is strategic as well as operational.

14 A strategic approach for statutory organisations

Summary

This chapter explores ways of building formal, ongoing and mainstream mechanisms, structures and cultures so that community involvement becomes an accepted, everyday part of the work of an organisation, and is integrated into all of its activities. This chapter will explore mechanisms which have been developed by both NHS organisations and local authorities (primarily social services) and also joint mechanisms. It also explores methods and approaches for reaching out to and involving services users, carers and local communities. Case studies are used to illustrate ways in which organisations have gone about trying to involve local people strategically, the difficulties and dilemmas identified, and some of the practical ways forward that have emerged from this work.

Introduction

Most of the chapters in this book have looked at ways of getting people involved in their own local communities, and in events and activities which are relevant to them as users of particular services. Clearly work and support that helps people to recognise and develop their skills, knowledge and confidence, and to see their own experiences as valid, is important. The ability of local communities to recognise common agendas, provide support and in some cases services for themselves, and work together for change is also important. However, this particular chapter is concerned with the other end of the participation spectrum; that is, the structures and mechanisms within organisations that can allow for effective participation in influencing decision making, priority setting and policies with organisations.

The 'onion' model: the layers needed to get to organisational participation

A few years ago this issue was discussed intensively at a weekend retreat held in Sheffield by the UK Health For All Network Community Participation Sub-Group. The group members coined the phrase 'organisational participation' to signify the process of communities (be they geographical or communities of interest) directly linking in to organisations. The following diagram was also developed at that same workshop to try and help people explore the links between community participation and community development. Community development was seen as a process for helping individuals, particularly people who were often excluded from the existing ways that people can make their views known, to move from a position of isolated individuals to the development of a collective, organised voice. Community participation was seen as a way of ensuring that that voice

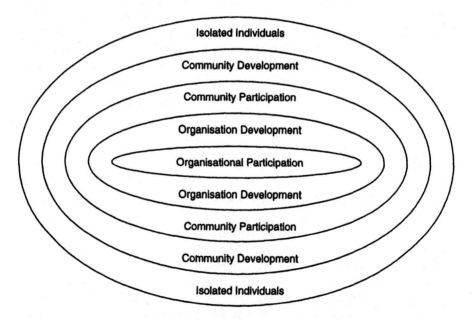

Figure 14.1   The 'onion' model of participation and development

could be fed through to decision and policy makers. Organisation participation was seen as a way of ensuring that there were mechanisms for
people to operate within the existing or purpose-developed structures and
mechanisms of organisations, rather than always lobbying from the outside. A model known as 'the onion' was developed to represent this visu-
ally.

Not all community development will lead to community participation;
some of the outcomes of community development may simply result in the
community setting up and running its own groups and activities. Not all
organisation development will lead to organisational participation; it may
simply be about ensuring that the organisation works more effectively and
efficiently internally. Some people are already well organised into effective
campaigning and lobbying groups and could be placed in the community
participation layer of the 'onion' without any need for community development; however, even these groups will have trouble influencing change and
getting through to the organisational participation layer unless the organisations they are attempting to negotiate, and work in partnership with,
have undergone some organisation development work so that they are
more amenable to, and structurally capable of working in partnership with,
community representatives.

**Case Study: The 'onion' model in practice (North Manchester Self-
Advocacy Project)**

Within the community of people with learning difficulties, the following
example of activities undertaken at each level of the 'onion' by the North
Manchester Self-Advocacy Project (Labyrinth 1993a) gives a practical illustration of what is meant. The 'onion' model is not static, of course, and
activities move over time. For example, at the outset of the project in 1991
most people with learning difficulties living in North Manchester would
have been in the outer layer as far as having a voice about services and
policies relating to them were concerned.

After a couple of years the project, through community development
work, had established a number of self-advocacy groups relating to different service-providing organisations (for example, day centres, group homes,
training centres). Thus some people had become organised, through community development support, to be in the 'community participation' layer.

Work was also undertaken by the project, and by the people with learning difficulties themselves, to influence staff and decision makers in the
organisations mentioned above, but also in organisations with a wider

strategic brief such as social services and the health authority. This took the form of running training to develop awareness about both the needs, and the capabilities of people with learning difficulties. It also focused on looking at the current mechanisms for influencing decision making and priorities around services for people with learning difficulties, such as the Joint Care Planning Team. The ways that meetings were structured and run were felt to mitigate against the participation of people with learning difficulties themselves. The self-advocacy project had had to address some of these issues in the way it organised itself; for example, the whole way management committee meetings were organised and run, and the way information was presented, had to be changed so that people with learning difficulties could actively participate in the management of their own project.

A Manchester 'People First' was established from the different advocacy groups supported by the North Manchester Self-Advocacy Project and others operating elsewhere in the city. This gave people with learning difficulties their own mechanism for representation and participation, through the election of a group of representatives to link into the joint planning process.

Initially the representatives chose the 'shadow' rather than attend formal care planning and other mechanisms. That is, they met to consider the agenda beforehand, and to feed in their views on the issues up for discus-

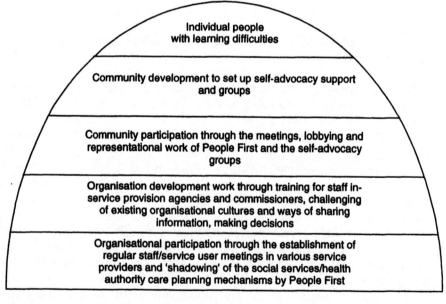

Figure 14.2   The 'onion' model in relation to North Manchester Self-Advocacy Project

sion, and afterwards commented on the minutes and decisions made at the meetings. Clearly the systems, structures and traditional professional ways of conducting meetings had not shifted sufficiently through the organisation development work to lead to full organisational participation for people with learning difficulties. This is hardly surprising given the scale of institutional change that would need to happen, and progress continues to be made.

Developing formal organisational strategies

The past couple of years have seen a growth of interest and practical work to produce organisational strategies in relation to community participation. Strategies are only useful if they lead to change and action, of course, but overall this must be regarded as a positive move as it ensures that organisations take more of a strategic rather than an *ad hoc* approach to community participation. It also allows for recognition of the complexity of moving from organisations that purchase for, or provide service to, people to organisations that purchase with or on behalf of people, and provide services based on expressed need rather than professional judgement alone.

Case Study: Sheffield Health Authority's Community Participation Strategy

Sheffield Health Authority is one of a small number of health authorities which have formally adopted a Community Participation Strategy. In the introduction to a summary version of the strategy called 'Involving the Public',[1] which was made available to local people in Sheffield, they state (p. 1):

We wish to involve local people more in the decisions we make. These include:

- How we spend the cash we get from Government on health services and on local health promotion work.
- What kinds of health services should be available.
- How services should be provided.
- How we change services so they are more in line with what local people need.

The strategy addresses ways of both taking forward and strengthening mechanisms and support for community participation and organisation development:

> Sheffield Health's core purpose is to assess needs, purchase quality services to meet needs and to develop ways to protect, improve and enhance health in the city.
>
> As part of this broad aim, Sheffield Health wishes to encourage and enable the views of Sheffield people, along with NHS staff and other agencies, to inform Sheffield Health's decision making about health promotion and health promotion and health services development and in its role as advocate for Sheffield people's health.
>
> Our objectives within this initiative are:
>
> - To develop a greater understanding of communities and agencies values in relation to health and health services.
> - To help inform people about Sheffield Health and health issues locally.
> - To listen to and take account of the needs and values of local people.
> - To establish mechanisms whereby we can enable communities views to be heard and inform Sheffield Health's work, decisions, priorities and resource allocation.
> - To ensure the views of all sections of the population are included in these processes, which will include acknowledging the value of advocacy as a process that will enhance community participation.
> - To evaluate our community participation processes and initiatives so we can make sure the methods we use are value for money.
> - To enhance health by promoting better understanding and participation in health issues.[2]

As well as providing a strategic framework for community participation and providing an action plan of work to be undertaken to begin turning the strategy into practice, the strategy document also highlights some key challenges. These are reproduced here, as they are likely to be issues that will need to be addressed or considered by a range of organisations and individuals involved in community participation at a strategic level:

> Trying to increase community participation is not an easy task. Some of the key challenges for Sheffield Health will be
>
> - Many groups and organisations will be involved in Sheffield Health's community participation work which will all have different expectations, and will have their own interests to pursue.
> - Expectations of the process and the capacity for Sheffield Health to change particular services, or use of resources quickly will be raised.
> - Sheffield Health will not always be able to respond as people would wish. There will be dilemmas to be faced, what if the government and local

people want different things, what if people and professionals want different things – whose views will predominate? We can overcome this by
being very clear from the outset with any piece of community participation work what we are trying to achieve, what scope we have for change,
how we will take on board what people want, what we cannot do and how
we will make decisions.

- People who have participated in organisations or consultations in the past
have often been middle class, white, male, literate and articulate and able
bodied. This is a stereotype, but often it *has* been a narrow section of the
population that has been able to participate. We need to encourage many
different kinds of people and interests to express their views and get
involved, not just the people who used to participate before the days of
community participation!

    In order to do this, we will need to undertake development work and
provide practical support.

- In order to enable CP, SH staff and other professionals such as GPs will
need to give up some of their professional power and listen and respond
to the views of local people. Some people will find this exciting and
others will find it threatening. Staff will need to be supported in this
work.

- For many years people have not been used to participating in public services, people have just received services (sometimes!) when they needed
them. It will take a cultural change and imaginative processes to encourage people to *want* to get involved. People will also need to believe it is
worthwhile and that they will be listened to.

- Questions of health and what impacts on it, what priority there should be
for treatments, who should be treated, what treatments should be provided, what should health policy concentrate on – all are very complex.
Often there are no 'right' answers and no 'experts', as issues are about
values and how we wish to act as a society. The HA is not ducking its
responsibilities in seeking public views over decisions to be made, it is
widening its sphere of influence and putting difficult questions into the
public arena for debate, rather than bureaucrats just making decisions
behind closed doors.

- The government policy is to create a primary health care led NHS and GPs
are key decision makers now as well as SH about health policy and use of
NHS resources. The GPs' first responsibility is to their patients. They have
not traditionally been professionally focused on communities' and
population's health (though many of course have an interest in this). There
are dilemmas for GPs and PHC teams in extending their role towards
more broadly based consultation with communities in case there are conflicts of views re patient and community needs. In addition for GPs in the
poorest areas of Sheffield the GP practice is often one of only a few local
agencies people can go to as other services may have disappeared. Although it is good a practice is a focal point in a community, many practices
cannot cope with the additional demands on their resources for essentially

social, economic and environmental needs and so may be reluctant to raise expectations further.

SH needs to support GPs and PHC staff in this process and enable development across the board in localities by working closely with other agencies to regenerate areas and redevelop local infrastructures and capacities.[3]

Other organisations such as Bradford Health Authority and South and West Devon Health Authority have also produced community development strategies. The latter used discussion of its document in draft form as a way of bringing together other key agencies and the voluntary sector to look at ways of producing a joint multi-agency CD and health strategy for each district council geographical area.

Methods and approaches to getting public involvement

In a study undertaken by one of the authors of this book (Labyrinth 1996b), a wide range of consultation and involvement mechanisms and structures was found to be in use by health authorities in England. These included:

- Sending documents out to community and voluntary groups for consultation.
- Focus groups.
- Citizens' juries.
- Health panels.
- Development of Neighbourhood Forums.
- Public meetings.
- Opening up of health authority meetings – style, access, venues.
- Regular use of the media.
- Production of accessible annual reports.
- Annual meetings open to the public.
- Questionnaires and surveys of different sorts – e.g. quality, satisfaction, qualitative, quantitative, structured, semi-structured, postal, face-to-face interviews, self-completion.
- Establishment of joint agency/community/user/carer working groups.
- Participatory needs assessment.
- Funding of community development work, advocacy initiatives, networks and forums.

Choice of methods or approach needs to take into account a number of factors. First is the focus on the word consultation (that is, a one-off seeking of views) or involvement (building an ongoing joint working partnership). Some methods are clearly more appropriate to the former than the latter.

The timescale that is being worked to is another important consideration. If a response is needed quickly then certain methods may be chosen in preference to ones that need a longer timescale to bring in ideas and information. However, this may be at the cost of building relationships and longer-term involvement. The resources available in terms of people, finances and in kind contributions will also affect your choice of methodology. It is important to have at least a broad idea of the costs involved before embarking on any particular approach. What is clear is that most of the approaches outlined above do have resource implications, to a greater or lesser extent.

People's level of knowledge and involvement about ways that decisions are made, and structures and mechanisms within and between organisations, are important factors too. Simply having a token 'representative' on a committee or planning group is pointless if that person cannot comprehend the detail of what is going on, and thus cannot make an informed contribution. An approach that starts with building up knowledge, skills and confidence within a geographical community or a community of interest, and builds in support and networking for representatives may be slower but yield more effective results in the long term.

Finally, methods need to take into account people's literacy levels, and issues in relation to race, culture, gender, physical and sensory ability, age and so forth. This may affect the detailed planning as well as the choice of method. Some methods that may initially seem unlikely choices can in fact be very effective if proper planning and support is built in as this case study shows.

Case Study: Consulting 'vulnerable' older people in Camden, London

In the London borough of Camden, following a number of local horrifying incidents, Camden Social Services and other partner agencies set out to consult 'vulnerable' older people about why some elderly people living in the borough rejected help from community services. They also wanted to seek older people's advice and involvement in improving the ways community services were planned and delivered. A small steering group was formed; it included a number of older people drawn from various groups, organisations and establishments. They were insistent that the best way to get a good cross-section of views, and to widen involvement, was to hold a day-long workshop for 'vulnerable' older people as well as undertaking discussions with people in their homes. As Camden has a multicultural population the needs of different communities also had to be built into the workshop organisation to ensure good levels of participation from older people from different communities. The workshop was a mammoth task to organise in terms of choice of venue, style of the sessions, transport, food, interpreters, publicity, help and support on the day, communication aids, and much more.

The day was a great success and was attended by a wide variety of older people, many with disabilities or who would usually be defined as 'housebound'. The workshop led to ongoing consultation and involvement work as well as some important initial ideas for services to take on board. A workshop might not have seemed the most logical or appropriate method to choose for this particular group of people; however, the advice of the older people on the steering group proved that professionals do not always know best! (see Labyrinth 1994c, 1995i).

Co-ordination and development work

In a follow-up study for the NHS Executive (Labyrinth 1993b), one year after the launch of the *Local Voices* document, the researchers found that health authorities took a different approach to the development and co-ordination of 'local voices' work . For example:

- By working through an existing structure or policy relating to community participation such as Health For All/Healthy Cities.
- By giving the lead to a particular part of the organisation, e.g. Communications, Public Health.
- By funding development workers within the voluntary sector.
- By employing/re-deploying a specialist worker with the authority itself.
- By including the lead within an individual's wider brief.
- By establishing a corporate cross-organisational team.
- By establishing a multi-agency team to work with the authority and wider.
- By the Chief Executive taking the lead.

- By delegating to each locality managers (where such an approach has been adopted by an authority.

This illustrates how the fifth element of the 'five elements for community involvement' (co-ordination and overview), which was explored in the previous chapter, has been put into practice by some health authorities.

The role of providers

Although the lead on public involvement and consultation was firmly allied to health authorities in the original *Local Voices* document (NHSME 1992b), clearly provider organisations also have a significant role to play in promoting and developing public consultation and involvement, as do GPs and other primary health care workers who now play an increasingly influential role in determining the allocation of NHS resources through fundholding, total purchasing initiatives and GP commissioning groups and now Primary Care Groups.

Community involvement can be built in to the role of providers in a number of ways. Some of these are initiatives that could be encouraged (or indeed required) by purchasers:

- Encourage positive attitudes to complaints, satisfaction surveys, etc., so that providers and purchasers can form a partnership to assess how services can be improved and developed.
- Explore with providers the impact of poor-quality services, or alienating styles of service delivery, of people's willingness to get involved and give their views, for example, are the majority of people less likely to give their views if they feel they are not listened to in service provision situations?
- Build community development and community involvement into contract specifications.
- Work to support and develop the provider capacity of voluntary and community organisations, and seek to contract with them.
- Provide or encourage training and staff development programmes (ideally multi-agency/multi-disciplinary) to build up skills in community involvement at all levels in agencies.

Involving service users and carers

The first part of this chapter has concentrated on strategic approaches from within the NHS. Community care has meant that the NHS must work in partnership with local authorities and the independent sector to look for ways of working together in terms of involving service users and carers. However, the ideas here could apply equally to 'patients' in services which the NHS is solely responsible for, as well as within community care.

The shift to 'community-based' care policy brought with it a duty upon agencies involved in the commissioning and delivering of services (and in particular social services as the lead co-ordinating agency) to consult and involve service users and carers. To move from a situation where tradition-ally most people were simply recipients of care to becoming active partners in determining needs and priorities requires radical change.

The first few years of the 1990s saw the establishment of a national initiative, 'Developing Managers for Community Care'.[4] The programme was set up in advance of the formal starting date for community care in April 1993, and ran on for some time afterwards as its aim was to support the transition as effectively as possible by developing the skills and apti-tudes of managers in all key agencies.

The programme consisted of a series of national networking and train-ing events, and the publication of around a dozen packs of materials and resources for people involved in management development and training work with NHS, Social Services and other key players in community care.

The scale and complexity of community care meant that organisations and individuals within them would need to be able to identify blocks and barriers, and to have the skills and aptitude to drive forward changes. The requirement for real, effective inter-agency working and the emphasis on service users' and carers' consultation and involvement were perceived as amongst the biggest challenges.

One area of focus was 'change management'. Early experience of com-munity care had shown that successful changes in community care require:

- A champion or leader providing energy, direction and vision.
- Effective people in key roles in each agency.
- A history of good, effective inter-agency working.
- A project manager who is empowered by the support and commitment of senior and operational managers across the agencies involved.
- A small, effective inter-agency group.
- Involvement of users and their representatives.
- Wide consultation with those who will be affected by the changes.

- Good communication up, down and across agencies.
- An internal or external facilitator with good content knowledge, process and inter-agency working skills.
- Financial and time resources to invest in development.
- Capacity to learn together and turn learning into action. [Dearden Management Ltd 1993]

Individuals charged with implementing changes need the following characteristics:

- A tolerance of uncertainty and lack of clear guidance.
- A liking for networking.
- A wide repertoire of interpersonal skills.
- Leadership qualities and influence skills.
- Analytical tools.
- Flexibility and staying power.
- Cross-agency knowledge. [Dearden Management Ltd 1993]

Involving Users & Carers in Inter-Agency Management Development (NHSTD 1993a) is a resource pack consisting of three development programmes. One focuses on developing the manager/user relationship; a second looks at partnerships with carers; the third consists of an outline programme and exercises for a search conference looking at developing local services for people. The materials are aimed at helping to maximise the involvement of users and carers in service planning and delivery by helping managers and professionals to:

- Develop a greater awareness of users and carers.
- Clarify language and meaning.
- Enable all participants to better understand each other's respective roles and responsibilities.
- Review obstacles to change.
- Consider how change should and can occur.
- Establish what action is needed locally to ensure services are user- and carer-led.

This broad checklist remains a useful basis for both starting work and monitoring progress in relation to service user and carer involvement.

A commitment to empowerment of service users and carers is a commitment to innovation. A pluralist strategy is needed to accommodate the different groups and individuals who seek services. Authority-wide initiatives within such a strategy might include:

- Development of customer contracts specifying the service to which the customer is entitled, standards and means of redress.
- User and citizen involvement in determining such standards and services.
- Statements of users' rights and how they can be enforced.
- Publication of information to assist choice.
- Effective complaints systems.
- Inspection of public and private activities.
- Development of quality audits.
- Creation of local and community forums and review bodies.
- Development of advocacy.
- Clarity about how the authority learns from the public and how it feeds back learning. [NHSTD 1994]

Good practice in care management can include:

- Asking users if they are happy with the service provided.
- Arranging feedback sessions involving users, carers and families.
- Using complaints and representations procedure as a constructive mechanism.
- Using appropriate language.
- Implementing equal opportunities policies/procedures.
- Doing assessment with the client and/or carer.
- Ensuring that all relevant views are taken into account in assessment.
- Providing information and honesty to the client about process and disclosure.
- Enabling the client to feel safe, secure and at ease.
- Ensuring user participation in the development of new services.
- Bringing in users as trainers for workers.
- Promoting information-giving, equality, accessibility.
- Keeping services under review. [NHSTD 1994]

Chapter 7 of this book explored the development of advocacy and the growth of service user and carer groups and networks. Parallel to this 'bottom up'-type development, some statutory organisations have developed user and care strategies

It is clear that a great deal of work is under way in relation to the involvement of users and carers, and that the last few years have seen significant changes in policy, planning, attitudes and services as a result of that involvement. Experience from around the country also strongly indicates that user and carer involvement needs to be considered separately.

There are a number of reports and publications which seek both to map activity and thinking, and to determine good practice. For example, in 1995 the Social Services Inspectorate (SSI) published a survey of local authorities in the North of England (SSI 1995). They found that, based on self-rating, most local authorities said they were a little better able to offer people care suitable to their needs; just under a third said they were much better, relative to pre-April 1993. Effective operation of systems and development of services were most often mentioned as criteria for evaluating success; user (and sometimes carer) satisfaction surveys were also mentioned, as were complaints. (Some said low levels of complaints indicated success, others said high numbers of complaints indicated success!)

A minority of local authorities mentioned autonomy as a priority in their new systems. Advocacy was mentioned by some as a means of empowerment. Self-assessment was cited as potentially liberating, and the making of payments to users through trusts or voluntary organisations is also highlighted.

Dilemmas and weaknesses were focused around the build-up of expectations which could not be met. The report noted there was still much to be done to meet the specific care and information and involvement needs of ethnic minority communities.

The methods of canvassing users' views which were most often mentioned were:

- Consultation during assessment.
- Satisfaction surveys.
- Complaints systems.
- Monitoring arrangements.

In a similar self-rating exercise by local authorities in relation to their support to carers, a minority said there had been no change in their support to carers; over two-thirds said they were a little better able to offer support to carers; and just under a third said they offered much better support (relative to pre-April 1993).

At that point between a quarter and a third of local authorities in the North offered separate assessment to carers (this percentage is likely to have increased significantly due to subsequent policy changes which stressed the need to assess carers separately from service users' needs).

False hopes of help were said to be leading to a drop-off in numbers of carers attending reference groups in some parts of the North. In some areas identification of carers was said to be difficult and, consequently, it was difficult to assess their needs. Dilemmas include lack of strategic thinking

and lack of practical planning about how to deal with differences of opinion between carers and users.
Ways of involving carers included:

- As trainers.
- In selecting staff.
- By more and better information, more widely displayed.
- Development of new services (e.g. more flexible respite care).
- In decision-making forums.

A survey amongst service planners, providers and users, to look at involving people in social services, was undertaken in 1990 (Croft and Beresford 1990). Although this research is now several years old, the findings remains pertinent to today's multi-sector community care scenario. Key findings from survey were:

- Policies and strategies for involving people are increasing.
- Involvement is both feasible and crucial.
- Increasing involvement of people in social services has resource implications (time and money), but does not necessarily mean more expensive services as it may also lead to savings in some areas and more effective provision overall.
- It is important to be clear about why people are being involved, and to what end, i.e. have clear objectives.
- There is a need to establish principles and guidelines for effective policy and practice.
- Progress on involvement is limited by lack of information and awareness.
- There is a need for improved and accessible information to help with informed decision making and choice.
- There has been a rapid increase in the numbers of user and self-advocacy organisations, but inadequate resources remain a major problem for such groups and organisations.
- There are two important components for effective involvement: access (structures and opportunities), and support (encouragement, confidence and skills).
- Two competing philosophies are operating: consumerism and self-advocacy; it is important to distinguish between the two.
- Involvement initiatives are more likely to be successful if workers and trade unions are also actively involved in developing them.
- It is important to access members of ethnic minorities and develop specific initiatives to involve them.

Croft and Beresford (1990) found that there was a wide range of levels of activity where there was involvement:

- Policy development.
- Service planning.
- Inspection.
- Quality.
- Research.
- Monitoring and evaluation.
- Assessment.
- Development and provision of own services and support packages.
- Advocacy.
- Complaints procedures.
- Access to records.

The survey identified the main ways in which people were involved in the running of existing services and the planning of new ones. Croft and Beresford ranked the responses in order of how often they were mentioned. Advisory groups, committees and forums were most often mentioned, followed by user/self-advocacy groups and committees. Management, steering groups and committees came next highest, followed by consultation meetings and finally planning, project work and service development groups.

Part of the survey sought to identify the problems people had encountered with involving people. These were looked at from both the perspective of service users and local people and of agencies. Both groups were also asked to suggest or explain ways that they had overcome difficulties.

For service users and local people the main problems were:

- Practical and personal obstacles (e.g. vulnerability, stress).
- People's lack of awareness or interest.
- Conflict between groups.
- 'Unrepresentativeness'.
- Lack of credibility.

Suggestions for ways of dealing with the difficulties service users and local people encountered were:

- Advocacy (citizen and self).
- Support groups.
- Training.
- Improved information.
- Improved access to agencies.

- Openness to, and support for, ideas and proposals.
- Clerical and administrative support.
- Payment of expenses.

The agencies interviewed highlighted different problems with involving people, though there are some similarities with the service users and local people's views above:

- Agency and/or staff resistance to involvement.
- Challenge to existing ways of doing things ('to' rather than 'with').
- Lack of skills.
- Past failures.
- Tokenism.
- Lack of time and resources.
- People's assumptions and/or lack of knowledge about agencies.

Agencies' ideas about ways of dealing with difficulties were also somewhat different, though also probably complementary rather than contradictory to service users' and local people's ideas:

- Clear terms of reference and objectives.
- Training and support for staff.
- Increased agency commitment.
- Funding of development workers.
- Developing a range of appropriate forums and opportunities for involvement.

Croft and Beresford (1990) drew up a list of guidelines for involvement (drawn from experience of both being service users themselves, and researchers in the community care field):

- Clarify what kind of involvement is on offer.
- Involve people from the start.
- Make clear the limits of involvement.
- Provide safeguards for people's involvement.
- Set small but attainable goals for change.
- Build people's participation into agency structures and functioning.
- Establish a continuing process of involvement.
- Develop anti-discriminatory forums and forums for involvement (not just traditional structures).
- Allow people's involvement to be flexible and open-ended.
- Ensure involvement is by choice not compulsion.

- Involve all the key participants concerned.
- Give priority to people's own accounts of their wants and needs.

A framework for involvement in community care

What emerges from the studies outlined above is the need to approach user and carer involvement strategically. There is also a degree of consensus that user and carer involvement needs to be seen, and taken forward, within a wider framework of public and community involvement.

The sections that follow suggest a number of models which can be used as both planning and review aids, which taken together can provide a framework for service user and carer involvement.

Breadth of support and development work

The list below seeks to set out the breadth of support and development work that is needed to take forward a comprehensive, strategic approach to user and carer involvement. It also gives examples of the sorts of initiatives that might be focused on (Labyrinth 1995d):

The breadth of support and development needed within a strategic approach to user and carer involvement is listed below (Labyrinth 1995d):

- General public e.g. building of a new 'care in the community' day care establishment in a particular locality; closure of a hospital-based service.
- All existing users and carers e.g. Community Care Plan Consultation; co-ordination of voluntary sector Joint Consultative Committee (JCC) input.
- All existing users e.g. User Involvement Forum; user involvement conference/event.
- All existing carers e.g. Carers' Centre; Carers' Strategy.
- Specific groups of users e.g. People First (learning difficulties); 'Hearing Voices' group (mental health).
- Specific groups of carers e.g. African-Caribbean carers; young carers.
- Carers of specific groups of people e.g. Parents in Partnership (learning difficulties); Carers of People with Alzheimer's Disease.
- Users of a specific service e.g. advocacy group in a day centre for people with learning difficulties; group home for people moved into the community from psychiatric hospital.

- Carers of people using a specific service   e.g. parents of young people with a learning difficulty living in a particular residential care establishment; carers of disabled people receiving respite care.
- Carers as service users in their own right   e.g. a Carers' Helpline; carers support group.
- Individual service user   e.g. own care plan; complaints procedures.
- Individual carer   e.g. own care/support plan; information pack.

At its widest, community care potentially involves all of us, that is, the general public. Many of us will be service users and/or carers in the future, even if we are not at the moment. Moving services out into the community has not happened without the community raising issues and concerns in relation to desirability, safety and so forth (even though much of the resistance has been based on stereotypes or inadequate information).

At its most specific, community care concerns individual carers and service users. However, not everyone who needs a service receives one at the moment, either because it is not suitable, because they do not know they are entitled to it, or perhaps because they are unhappy with the way in which it is delivered. So we cannot just rely on contacting and involving existing service users, it is also important to have a wider involvement perspective.

Levels of involvement

Figure 14.3 summarises some examples of the different levels of involvement that users and/or carers might be party to. At the top of the 'ladder' are services developed and run by users themselves, based on their own assessment of need.

Such self-determination is the ultimate in terms of involvement, although it may not be possible or desirable for all services to be provided by service users themselves (however, the Wiltshire case study which follows this section illustrates how successful such initiatives can be). The bottom of the ladder represents the traditional way that most services have been developed and run, with the user as a passive recipient rather than an active participant in the process. Other levels in between move from information giving, up to consultation, then to joint planning, and to direct involvement in management.

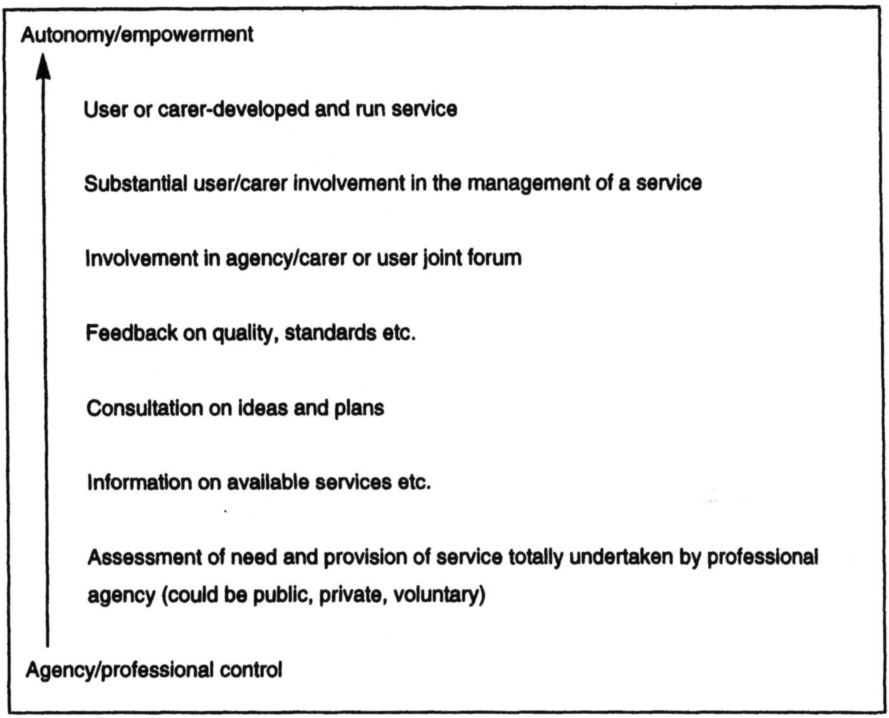

Autonomy/empowerment

↑

    User or carer-developed and run service

    Substantial user/carer involvement in the management of a service

    Involvement in agency/carer or user joint forum

    Feedback on quality, standards etc.

    Consultation on ideas and plans

    Information on available services etc.

    Assessment of need and provision of service totally undertaken by professional agency (could be public, private, voluntary)

Agency/professional control

Figure 14.3   Levels of involvement and participation (Labyrinth 1995d)

Areas for development and change

The process of bringing about change to increase and strengthen user and carer involvement in community care needs to operate within separate but linked areas (see Figure 14.4, adapted from Figure 13.1 'Five elements of a community involvement strategy'). Some of the required changes will be in relation to the individual carer or service user. This might be brought about by increased awareness of rights, through more information, individual support, access to new services or improvements in existing services, increases in confidence, or advocacy. Equally, it might be brought about through anger at the lack of availability of appropriate services, through a complaint, or other sorts of self-directed motivation.

In the collective arena (that is, individual people coming together for a common purpose), change might be brought about by the establishment of a support group, an advocacy service, by obtaining funding for a user-managed service, training, consultation workshops, focus groups and so

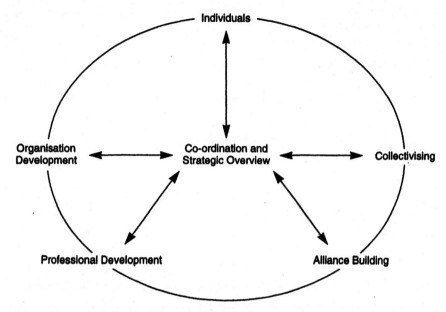

Figure 14.4   Levels of action and change in user and carer involvement (Labyrinth 1995d)

on. These may be initiated through agencies, or users or carers themselves, or jointly.

At the alliance-building level, groups of carers, or groups of users, may come together occasionally (for example, at a one-off event), or formally (for example, the self-advocacy groups for people with learning difficulties in North Manchester stimulated the setting up of a Manchester-wide People First organisation).

Change in relation to professional development may include managers and workers being given new opportunities to work in different ways, undergoing training to challenge attitudes, and learn new skills – because of the challenges of community care in general, and user and carer involvement in particular.

At the organisation development level, organisations providing services may have to radically change their culture, structures and systems in order to accommodate and take on board user and carer involvement. This may also involve changes in roles and responsibilities and new ways of working (for example, jointly with other organisations and agencies, and directly in partnership with user and carer groups).

Different approaches to strategic working

The case studies that follow set out some examples of strategic working in relation to service user and carer involvement taken by different organisations around the country. The first two are examples of where statutory funding has helped to build up and develop the voluntary sector and user and carer infrastructures in order to take forward partnership working. The latter two are examples of where research has been used to identify a strategic way forward based on need and the perspectives of service users and carers.

Case Study: Wiltshire Community Care User Involvement Network (WCCUIN)

WCCUIN is a Registered Company Limited by Guarantee. They are concerned with the empowerment of users and with direct involvement to bring about change. The organisation developed out of the first Wiltshire Community Care Consultation Conference held early in 1991. The organisation has grown substantially over that time, from a very small number of people to very wide involvement, and from an idea to running a company with a £250,000 budget.

The organisational infrastructure includes:

- The Planning Group – registered legal directors elected at the AGM. They meet approximately once every two months and are given training at the outset to learn about the organisation and their roles within it.
- The staff – initially in 1994, there were three permanent members of staff, by March 1995 there were 16. These include a director/convenor, a finance manager and assistant, an administration manager and two other admin staff, a development worker and two other outreach staff, a team of six people supporting the Wiltshire Independent Living Fund, and staff working on Living Options, Patients' Council and the Information Project.
- The different areas of the work are steered by advisory committees controlled by service users.

Most of the funding comes from statutory purchasers (for example, Social Services and Wiltshire Health Authority via their three-year rolling Service Level Agreement), though some also comes from trusts and other non-statutory sources. The organisation reaches out to new service users, provides regular information, supports user involvement, establishes rights groups, and reaches out to marginalised users.

WCCUIN is involved in direct action to bring about change in a range of areas:

- Developing and managing user-controlled services (Patients' Council Support Group, Wiltshire Independent Living Fund, Living Options Partnership Project, Wiltshire Information Federation, Salisbury Information Centre).
- Users taking the lead in policy development.
- Users influencing policy development.
- User involvement in information preparation.
- User involvement in the production of the Community Care Plan.
- User involvement in the development of Care Management.
- Links with the Social Services Inspection Unit.
- User involvement in training.
- User involvement in employment.
- User involvement in Performance and Quality Unit.
- Users in relation to transport.
- Users acting as a development agency.
- User involvement in research.
- Links with the voluntary sector.
- Meetings and workshops.
- Users at conferences.
- Involvement in health and health provision.
- Users' perspectives in housing strategy.
- Promoting good practice through advising, training, presentations, disseminating learning, publishing articles and media links, learning from user-controlled projects.

Case Study: Manchester Alliance for Community Care (MACC)

MACC is a small voluntary organisation that was originally initiated as a project within Voluntary Action Manchester but is now an independent voluntary organisation, with its own management committee. Funded through Joint Finance, it employs a development worker and an administrator, and also houses the voluntary sector's joint planning/commissioning worker.

MACC supports specific groups of service users, such as the 'Hearing Voices' (schizophrenia) Group, and also undertakes general co-ordination of user involvement into Manchester's various service planning, commissioning and providing agencies. The project helps support advocacy development, training, consultation and so forth.

The next case study is an example of a needs assessment exercise with carers undertaken by consultants working in West Lancashire (Hill and Nugent 1994). It illustrates how a strategic approach to needs assessment can result in very comprehensive framework for involvement and for meeting carers' needs.

Case Study: A strategic approach to looking at carers' needs in West Lancashire

This research was undertaken by outside consultants working to a steering group which included statutory services, voluntary organisations and carers. The main recommendations are summarised below under four main headings: identifying carers, involving carers, informing carers and supporting carers.

How to identify carers

- Establish a voluntary 'Register of Carers'.
- Assessment forms and procedures should be used as an opportunity for identification of, and communication with, carers.
- GP (via GP tutors) and primary health care training (HAs and Trusts) should include raising awareness of issues concerning carers.
- The role of pharmacists in assisting carers to identify themselves should be explored.

How to involve carers

- Views should be taken into account in any proposed changes to planning and delivery of community care.
- There should be a minimum of two carers on any committee.
- Resources should be available to ensure that 'representative' carers can be in communication with, and accountable to, other carers.

- Carers should be paid for their consultancy or training expertise and paid travel and sitting expenses.
- Use existing and establish new carer-led self-help groups.
- Organise training for managers in:

    - consulting with carers;
    - sharing decision making with carers; and
    - planning and managing change.

- Organise training for staff in:

    - stereotyping of carers;
    - communicating with carers; and
    - listening to carers.

How to inform carers and keep them informed

- Develop a creative information campaign to get the message out to carers and professionals about services and resources tailored to carers' needs.
- Produce a simple leaflet about proposed new carers' service (Carers' Resource Centre) and deliver it to every household.
- A free quarterly newsletter should be mailed to all on the Carers' Register, with inserts from all relevant agencies.
- Resource packs which include a range of information on services and support should be available for all carers.
- Inter-agency agreement is needed as to who will lead on providing advice on benefits.
- Each purchasing and providing organisation should have a named person responsible for co-ordinating carers' information and issues. This co-ordinating role should be included in the job descriptions and time allocated to carry out this role.

Supporting carers in their caring role

- Funding should be made available to establish and run a Carers' Resource Centre offering:

    - a range of relevant training for carers;
    - a telephone help line;
    - counselling;
    - outreach;
    - newsletter; and
    - provision of specialist advice.

- A flexible all-night respite care service should be provided.
- Action for carers should be recognised as part of the formal planning machinery.
- Services available to carers should be marketed.
- Local branch of the Carers' National Association should be properly funded (for adequate worker time and premises).
- GPs, Trusts and Health Authorities should promote self-help carers' groups and offer meeting space in health centres, and so on.
- Support services should not cease just because the person is no longer formally caring for someone – they should continue as long as the carer feels they need them.
- Carers receiving community care services should be visited, or at least telephoned, at specific intervals to demonstrate support and enquire about changes in circumstances.

Case Study: A strategic approach to looking at carers' needs in Tameside

The final case study is based on work undertaken in Tameside (Watters 1995). This work focused particularly on the needs of carers in the Home Care service; it was part of a wider joint multi-agency strategy for carers. The research was intended to develop good practices for carer involvement right at the start of the Carers' Strategy. It has also influenced general thinking on carer involvement in relation to the Community Care Planning process and 'customer care' in general in the various agencies.

The specific aims of this project were to involve carers to look at four key areas:

- Carers' access to services.
- Carers being involved in decisions.
- Carers having their own needs recognised by others.
- Carers recognising themselves as carers.

The Home Care service was chosen as a specific focus as this was the most common form of service delivery, apart from GPs, with which carers had contact.

The project objectives were:

- To look specifically at the needs of carers in the way the Home Care service is assessed and delivered.

- To identify ways carers can be involved in service planning and assessment, and the assessment and recognition of their own needs.
- To identify difficulties which may exist for ethnic minority carers and families.
- To test out 'best practice' ideas and models in a specific locality.
- To use the findings to support the separate needs of carers and anti-discriminatory practice.

The 1985 General Household Survey defined a carer as someone who was 'looking after, or providing some regular service for, someone who was sick, elderly or handicapped', either in their own household or elsewhere. Tameside Council's definition is, 'anyone whose life is restricted by the continuing need to care for a family member or friend who is frail, ill or has a disability'.

The researchers initially looked at national literature sources and identified the most common areas of need for carers that emerged from other studies. These were:

- Information and advice.
- Financial.
- Practical help.
- Housing.
- Respite.
- Emotional and social support.
- Recognition of minority groups.

The research looked at carers' needs (in Tameside) in relation to each of the above. Their conclusions and recommendations are summarised below:

- Information provision to be reviewed to better meet the needs of carers in relation to the following:

  - quality and methods of provision;
  - promotion of self-recognition amongst carers;
  - informing professionals, especially GPs, and using them as an information resource;
  - complaints procedures; and
  - consultation about information provision.

- Recommendations/issues for consideration in relation to assessment:

  - separate assessment for carers and users;
  - assessment to be needs-led and pro-active by carers;

- more extensive, integrated, pro-active assessment process for carers;
- possible role of carers' advocates; and
- improved reassessment procedures.

• The following areas were identified as in need of review in relation to the performance of the Home Care Service:

- amount of time provided;
- flexibility of timing;
- flexibility of tasks performed;
- dependability; and
- training and advice to carers.

• The following areas were identified as in need of review in relation to minority groups:

- information needs; and
- performance against special needs.

• The following were identified as in need of review in relation to service planning and resource issues:

- collaboration within and between agencies;
- individually based, needs-led service planning;
- prioritisation; and
- role of the independent sector.

Notes

1 Sheffield Health Authority Community Participation Strategy, 'Involving the Public', Executive Summary, 1997.
2 Ibid. p. 7.
3 Ibid. pp. 20–21.
4 'Developing Managers for Community Care' was a national programme, managed by the NHS Management Executive and the Social Services Inspectorate, which ran from 1991 to 1994 and produced around a dozen publications (published by the NHS Training Directorate (now Division) in Bristol).

15 Conclusions

Our aim in writing this book is to make visible some of the history and achievements, as well the trials and tribulations, of all those individuals, groups, organisations, networks and movements who have worked to make sure that they have some involvement in their own health and some control over the issues, decisions and conditions that affect their health and the health of the wider community. We hope that the material in this book illustrates this process in all its contradictions, describing the factors which have enabled great strides to be made forward, as well as those which have inhibited progress. Crucially, too, our aim is to describe some of the models, strategies, interesting case studies and practical checklists for action that have been developed and can be used by those active in the field, to build on and take forward existing achievements.

It seems that right now conditions are such in the UK that our historic achievements can be built on, and lessons learnt can be capitalised on. However, for this to be so, some of the gaps revealed in the movement to take forward community involvement in health must be filled. Also, the potential and opportunities for progress must be realised. We argue here that these must be addressed locally and nationally, by those at all levels of government, organisations and communities.

Our work has revealed at least four main gaps that need to be plugged for progress to be made. First, the embryonic networks of those interested in community development approaches to health must be supported and resourced; the community health movement needs the involvement of those active in the field as well as the commitment of top policy makers. This message has met with more recent success in Scotland, Northern Ireland and Wales than in England. The first three countries each have some form of community health network (though in Wales it operates through a statutory agency rather than independently, and has more limited functions). In England the Community Development and Health Network (England) was launched at a national conference in Oldham in September 1997, after two years of regional, local and national networking between people active in the field. However, it has yet to be successful in gaining funds. Resourcing of such networks is not an expensive business. The principles of community development suggest that structures which take their lead from the field, employing a few workers to take on development, information and co-ordination tasks, are more effective in sustaining effective networking than top-heavy national 'centres'.

Second, community development and health theories, models and practice need to be built into mainstream professional training of health workers at all levels, including general practitioners, public health doctors, community nurses, health promotion specialists and so on. Otherwise such approaches, aimed at moving people from being 'passive recipients' of health services to 'active participants' in their own health, will remain marginalised and fringe activities.

Third, there needs to be a more active linking of community development approaches with organisation development approaches. We argue in this book that the principles and methods used in these two approaches are remarkably similar. In practice, when they are brought together, great gains are made as community involvement in health can then become sustainable. Such linkage allows progress on health issues to be made within communities, while also addressing the need to examine and change organisational structures and mechanisms which may inhibit ongoing community involvement at different levels. It would help managers within the health service to make connections between the theories and practice of participatory styles of management, and those of community development in health.

In addition, there is still a gap between the advocacy movement and the community health movement within the UK. The principles and practices of each are very similar; it is the constituents which tend to vary. Advocacy tends to be used among 'service users and carers', especially in a community care context, while community development tends to be used among geographic communities or communities of interest. Making the links between the two would be of benefit as it would allow a more efficient use of resources, and for sharing of ideas, progress and actions. National networking would help to encourage such linkage locally. We know of one area (Calderdale) which has consciously sought to establish such links by setting up a Partnership Project supported by the local authority, health authority and voluntary sector, which aims to establish the fullest possible involvement of users, carers and the voluntary sector in joint planning at all levels of the local authority and health authority, but equally take in community development, health promotion and community regeneration initiatives.

There is potential and opportunity for progress to be made in community involvement in health. We are moving towards a primary health care-led NHS and this has sparked off considerable interest in the use of community development approaches within primary care settings, and indeed the work of the Public Health Alliance Trust's Primary Care Project suggests that CD is in fact an integral part of primary care in itself. It is important that this policy and practice shift does not seek to 'reinvent the wheel' but instead builds on the lessons of the recent past, such as the *Local Voices* initiative and Health For All as well as the community health movement. It is interesting in this connection that the 4th International Conference on Health Promotion held in 1997 in Jakarta reaffirmed the importance of community participation as a key element of Health For All. At the same time the current government climate is positive regarding community involvement and health. The Labour government has for the first time appointed a Minister for Public Health and is making stronger linkages between a new public health policy and the funding of economic regeneration initiatives.

Finally, then, we are fortunate in the UK to have a considerable history and developed expertise in the field of community involvement in health. Through the recent legacy of *Local Voices*, community care and so on, statutory organisations are now at least aware of the need to consult and involve local communities, and some are doing much more to bring this about. Therefore we have the conditions for strong and successful 'bottom up/top down' partnerships in health. All that is missing, it seems, is a strong policy connection and national networking between these two levels.

Appendix: Useful organisations

ACRE (Action for Communities in Rural England)
Dean House, Somerford Court, Somerford Road, Cirencester GL7 1TW
Tel: 01285 653 477

ACW (Association of Community Workers)
Stephenson Building, Elswich Road, Newcastle NE4 6SQ
Tel: 0191 281 4419

ACHCEW (Association of Community Health Councils for England and Wales)
30 Drayton Park, London N5 1PB
Tel: 0171 609 8405   Fax: 0171 700 1152

Association of Metropolitan Authorities (now Local Government Association)
26 Chapter House Street, London SW1P 4ND
Tel: 0171 834 2222

BASSAC (British Association of Settlements and Social Action Centres)
1st Floor, Winchester House, 11 Cranmer Road, London SW9 6EJ
Tel: 0171 735 1075

Churches' Community Work Alliance
36 Sandygate, Wath-on-Dearne, Rotherham, S63 7LW
Tel: Not known

CDF (Community Development Foundation)
60 Highbury Grove, London N5 2AG
Tel: 0171 226 5375

CDH Network (England)
c/o SCCD, 356 Glossop Road, Sheffield S10 2HW
Tel: 0114 270 1718

CDH Network (Northern Ireland)
Ballybot House, 22 Cornmarket, Newry BT35 8BG
Tel: 01693 64606

CDH Network (Scotland)
Suite 329, Baltic Chambers, 50 Wellington Street, Glasgow G2 6HJ
Tel: 0141 248 1924

Community Health UK
6 Terrace Walk, Bath BA1 1LN
Tel: 01225 462680   Fax: 01225 484238

Community Links
237 London Road, Sheffield S2 4NF
Tel: 0114 258 8822   Fax: 0114 255 9595

Community Matters
8/9 Upper Street, London N1 0PQ
Tel: 0171 226 0189   Fax: 0171 354 9570

CORU (Community Operational Research Unit)
Northern College, Wentworth Castle, Stainborough, Barnsley S75 3ET
Tel: 01226 285 426   Fax: 01226 284 308

Drumchapel Community Health Project
Drumchapel Health Centre, 80–90 Kinfauns Drive, Glasgow G15 7TX
Tel: 0141 211 6166

Faculty of Community Medicine
4 St Andrews Place, Regents Park, London NW1 4LB
Tel: 0171 935 0035

FCWTG (Federation of Community Work Training Groups)
356 Glossop Road, Sheffield S10 2HW
Tel: 0114 273 9391

Greater Chesterton Community Programme (now Chesterton Community
Partnership)
Chesterton Community Office, 6 Edensor Court, London Road, Chesterton,
Newcastle, Staffs. ST5 7EA
Tel: 01782 562003

Healthy Alliance Team
Health Promotion Department
North Staffordshire Health Authority
Herbert Minton Building, 79 London Road, Stoke on Trent, Staffs. ST4 7PZ
Tel: 01782 744444

HEBS (Health Education Board for Scotland)
Woodburn House, Canaan Lane, Edinburgh EH10 4SG
Tel: 0131 447 8044   Fax: 0131 452 8140

Hutson Street Project
4 Dunoon House, Newall Street, Bradford BD5 7QA
Tel: 01274 390097

King's Fund
11–13 Cavendish Square, London W1M 0AN
Tel: 0171 307 2400

MACC (Manchester Alliance for Community Care)
Swan Buildings, 20 Swan Street, Ancoats, Manchester M4 5JW
Tel: 0161 834 9823

NACVS (National Association of Councils for Voluntary Services)
3rd Floor, Arundel Court, 177 Arundel Street, Sheffield S1 2NU
Tel: 0114 278 6636

NCVO (National Council for Voluntary Organisations)
Regent's Wharf, 8 All Saint's Street, London N1 9RL
Tel: 0171 713 6161   Fax: 0171 713 7300

NHS Confederation (previously NAHAT)
Birmingham Research Park, Vincent Drive, Birmingham B15 2SQ
Tel: 0121 471 4444

Organisation Development Network (England)
c/o Aspire Consultants, 1st Floor, 299 Ecclesall Road, Sheffield S11 8NX
Tel: 0114 268 0814

People First
207–215 King's Cross Road, London WC1X 9DB
Tel: 0171 713 6400

PHA (Public Health Alliance)
BVSC, 138 Digbeth, Birmingham B5 6DR
Tel: 0121 643 4343/7628   Fax: 0121 643 4541   E-mail: pht@ukonline.co.uk

Salford Community Health Project
Higher Broughton Health Centre, Bevenden Square, Salford M7 4TF
Tel: 0161 792 6969

SCCD (Standing Conference for Community Development)
356 Glossop Road, Sheffield S10 2HW
Tel: 0114 270 1718   Fax: 0114 276 2377

UKHFAN (Health For All Network (UK) Ltd.)
PO Box 101, Liverpool L69 5BE
Tel/Fax: 0151 207 0919

WCCUIN (Wiltshire Community Care User Involvement Network)
7 Prince Maurice Court, Hambleton Avenue, London Road, Devizes
SH10 2RT
Tel: 01380 725213

Wells Park Health Project
1 Wells Park Road, Sydenham, London SE26 6JE
Tel: 0181 699 2840   Fax: 0181 699 2552

West Bowling Community Health Action Project
Community Action Station, Ryan Street, Bradford BD5 7AS
Tel: 01274 738645

Bibliography

Adams, L. (1991) 'Community development at a national level within the Health Education Authority', in *'Roots and Branches': Papers from the OU/ HEA 1990 Winter School on Community Development and Health*, Milton Keynes: Open University.

Adams, L. and Smithies, J. (1993) 'Walking the tightrope: Issues in evaluation and community participation for Health for All', in J. Davies and M. Kelly (eds) (1993) *Healthy Cities: Research and Practice*, London: Routledge.

Alinsky, S.D. (1972) *Rules for Rascals: A Pragmatic Primer for Realistic Radicals*, USA: Vintage.

Anyanwu, C.N. (1988) 'The technique of participatory research in community development', *Community Development Journal*, **23**, 1.

Association of Metropolitan Authorities (AMA) (1993) *Local Authorities and Community Development: A Strategic Opportunity for the 1990s*, London: Association of Metropolitan Authorities.

Batson, B. and Smith, J. (1995) *Organisational Development in the Community: Application, Tools and Discussion*, Occasional Papers in Social Studies, International Policy Research Unit, Leeds Metropolitan University; London: Community Development Foundation.

Beattie, A. (1991) 'The evaluation of community development initiatives in health promotion: A review of current strategies', in *'Roots and Branches': Papers from the OU/HEA 1990 Winter School on Community Development and Health*, Milton Keynes: Open University.

Beckhard, R. and Harris, R.T. (1987) *Organisational Transactions: Managing Complex Change*, Wokingham, Berks.: Addison-Wesley Publishing Co. (2nd edn).

Blennerhassett, S., Farrant, W. and Jones, J. (1989) 'Support for community health projects in the UK: A role for the National Health Service', *Health Promotion*, 4(3).

Bottomley, V. (10/9/1996) *Building Communities: Community Development, Participation and Partnership*, speech transcript, London: Department of National Heritage.

Bradford Health Authority (1995) *Bradford Health Authority CD Strategy*, internal document.

Brager, G. and Specht, H. (1973) *Community Organizing*, New York: Columbia University Press.

Brinberg, D. and McGrath, J.E. (1985) *Validity and the Research Process*, London: Sage.

Butler, K., Carr, S. and Sullivan, F. (1988) *Citizen Advocacy: A Powerful Partnership*, London: National Citizen Advocacy (now Citizen Advocacy Information and Training).

Caple, T. (1990) *Preparing People for Change: A Handbook for Trainers and Managers*, NHS Training Authority.

Chanan, G. (1991) *Taken For Granted: Community Activity and the Crisis of the Voluntary Sector*, London: Community Development Foundation Publications.

Chanan, G. (1992) *Community Development Monitoring Scheme*, London: Community Development Foundation (internal document).

CHIRU/LCHR (1987a) *Report of the First National Community Health Action Conference*, London: Community Health Initiatives Resource Unit, and London Community Health Resource.

CHIRU/LCHR (1987b) *Guide to Community Health Projects*, London: National Council for Voluntary Organisations.

Clark, E. (1995) *'Hear Me...': Advocacy in Surrey*, Thames Ditton: Surrey Social Services.

Coke, J. (1991), 'Building Alliances: But on Whose Terms – Some Reflections on a Black Woman's Experiences', in *'Roots and Branches'; Papers from the OU/HEA 1990 Winter School on Community Development and Health*, Milton Keynes: Open University.

Community Development Foundation and Labyrinth Training and Consultancy (1996) *Monitoring and Evaluation Scheme: Action Booklet*, Cardiff: Health Promotion Wales.

Community Links (1997) *Ideas Annual '97: A Guide to Good Ideas in Community Development and Health*, London: Community Links.

Craig, G. (1989) 'Community Work and the State', *Community Development Journal*, 24(1).

Croft, S. and Beresford, P. (1990) *From Paternalism to Partnership: Involving People in Social Services*, Open Services Project (London) and Joseph Rowntree Foundation (York).

Crombie, H. (1995) *Sustainable Development and Health*, Birmingham: Public Health Alliance.

Davies, J. and Kelly, M. (eds) (1993) *Healthy Cities: Research and Practice*, London: Sage.

Dearden Management Ltd (1993) *Care Management: Change Management*, Bristol: NHS Training Directorate.

Department of Health (1990) 'Local people must be involved in purchasing', press release.

Department of Health (1992) *The Health of the Nation: A Strategy for Health in England*, London: HMSO.

Department of Health (1993) *The Health of the Nation*, London: HMSO.

Department of Health (1997) *The New NHS. Modern. Dependable*, London: HMSO.

Department of Health (1998) *Our Healthier Nation*, London: HMSO.

Department of the Environment (1995) *Partners in Regeneration: Involving Communities in Urban and Rural Regeneration*, London: HMSO.

Department of the Environment (1997a) *SRB Challenge Fund Round 4: Supplementary Guidance*, London: HMSO.

Department of the Environment (1997b) *Single Regeneration Budget (SRB) Challenge Fund: Bidding Guidance, Round 4* (March).

DHSS(NI) (1996) *Health and Wellbeing: Into the Next Millennium*. Regional Strategy for Health and Social Wellbeing 1997–2002 (no date or place of publication).

Douglas, J. (1991) 'Influences on the Community Development and Health Movements – A Personal View', in *'Roots and Branches': Papers from the OU/HEA 1990 Winter School on Community Development and Health*, Milton Keynes: Open University.

Drumchapel CHP (Community Health Project) (1990) *Local Voices, Local Lives: The Story of the Kendoon Community Health Profile*. Video and report. Available from Drumchapel Health Centre, 80–90 Kinfauns Drive, Drumchapel, Glasgow G15 7TX.

Dunning, A. (1995) *Citizen Advocacy with Older People: A Code of Good Practice*, London: Centre for Policy on Ageing.

Ewles, L. and Simnett, I. (1992) *Promoting Health: A Practical Guide*, London: Scutari Press (2nd edn).

Farrant, W. (1991) 'Questioning the Contradictions: 'Health for All' and the Community Health Movement', in *'Roots and Branches': Papers from the OU/HEA 1990 Winter School on Community Development and Health*, Milton Keynes: Open University.

FCWTG (Federation of Community Work Training Groups) (1994) *Community Work: Scottish NVQ Project*.

Feuerstein, M.-T. (1986) *Partners in Evaluation: Evaluating Development and Community Programmes with Participants*, London: Macmillan.

Feuerstein, M.-T. (1988) 'Finding the methods to fit the people: Training for participatory evaluation', *Community Development Journal*, 23, 1: 16–25.

Finch, J. (1986) *Research and Policy: The Uses of Qualitative Methods in Social and Educational Research*, The Falmer Press.

Fordham, G. (1995) *Made to Last: Creating Sustainable Neighbourhood and Estate Regeneration*, York: Joseph Rowntree Foundation.

Freeman, R., Gillam, S., Shearin, C. and Pratt, J. (1997) *Community Development in Primary Care: A Guide to Involving the Community in COPC*, London: King's Fund.

French, W.L. and Bell, C.H. (1984) *Organisation Development*, Prentice Hall (3rd edn).

Funnell, R., Oldfield, K. and Speller, V. (1995) *Towards Healthier Alliances: A Tool for Planning, Evaluating and Developing Healthy Alliances*, London: Health Education Authority.

Gamble, D.N. and Weil, M.O. (1997) 'Sustainable development: the challenge for community development', *Community Development Journal*, 32(3), July.

Green, J. and Chapman, A. (1991) 'The Lessons of the Community Development Project for Community Development Today', in *'Roots and Branches': Papers from the OU/HEA 1990 Winter School on Community Development and Health*, Milton Keynes: Open University.

Green, J. and Price, D. (1996) *'It's called a health project...but they do a bit of all sorts there'*. An Evaluation of the Riverside Community Health Project: Summary Report (January), Social Welfare Research Unit, University of Northumbria.

Hanmer, J. (1991) 'The influence of feminism on Community Development and Health', in *'Roots and Branches': Papers from the OU/HEA 1990 Winter School on Community Development and Health*, Milton Keynes: Open University.

Health Education Authority (1992) *Partnerships in Health Promotion: Collaboration between the Statutory and Voluntary Sectors*, London: Health Education Authority.

HEC/THR (Health Education Council/Training in Health and Race) (1985) *Training in Health and Race: Final Report*, London: Health Education Council.

Health of the Nation (1993) *Working Together for Better Health*, London: Department of Health.

Health of the Nation (1995) *Variations in Health: What can the Department of Health Do?*, London: Department of Health.

Healthgain Conference (1992) *The Public as Partners: A Toolbox for Involving*

Local People in Commissioning Health Care, Cambridge: Healthgain Conference.

Healthy Sheffield Support Team (1993) *Community Development and Health: The Way Forward in Sheffield,* Sheffield: Health and Consumer Services, Sheffield Council.

Hill, G. and Nugent, P. (1994) *Carers in the Community in West Lancashire: Report of a Research Project into the Needs of Carers in West Lancashire,* West Lancashire Action for Carers.

Hunter, D. (1993) 'An opportunity to put health before health care', *Health Matters,* Spring, pp. 1–3.

Jones, J. (1991), 'Community Development and Health Education: Concepts and Philosophy', in *'Roots and Branches': Papers from the OU/HEA 1990 Winter School on Community Development and Health,* Milton Keynes: Open University.

Kanter, R.M. (1985) *The Change Masters: Corporate Entrepreneurs at Work,* London: Unwin.

Kenner, C. (1986) *Whose Needs Count? Community Action for Health,* Bath: Community Health UK.

Kilminster, S. (1996) *Hutson Street Health Project: An Evaluation,* Bradford: Hutson Street Project.

Kramarae, C. and Treichler, P. A. (1985) *A Feminist Dictionary,* London: Pandora Press.

Kunz, C., Jones, R. and Spencer, K. (1989) *Building for Change? Voluntary Organisations and Competitive Tendering for Local Authority Services,* Birmingham: Community Projects Foundation and Birmingham Settlement.

Labyrinth Training and Consultancy (1991) *Saltley Health Action Area: A Survey of Existing Reports, Studies and Information,* London: Labyrinth Training and Consultancy.

Labyrinth Training and Consultancy (1993a) *An Evaluation of the North Manchester Self-Advocacy Project,* for the Project; Haworth: Labyrinth Training and Consultancy.

Labyrinth Training and Consultancy (1993b) *Responding to Local Voices: An Overview of the Implications for Purchasing Organisations,* for the Purchasing Section, NHS Management Executive; Haworth: Labyrinth Training and Consultancy.

Labyrinth Training and Consultancy (1993c) *A Review of the Values and Benefits of 'Look After Yourself' Activities in Airedale, West Yorkshire,* for Airedale Health Authority; Haworth: Labyrinth Training and Consultancy.

Labyrinth Training and Consultancy (1993d) *Accessing the Views of Local People,* for Oldham Local Voices Steering Group and West Pennine Health Authority; Haworth: Labyrinth Training and Consultancy.

Labyrinth Training and Consultancy (1994a) *Community Involvement in Health: A Strategy for Kirkby*, for St Helens & Knowsley Health; Haworth: Labyrinth Training and Consultancy.

Labyrinth Training and Consultancy (1994b) *Speaking Out for Advocacy*, Conference Report, Haworth: Labyrinth Training and Consultancy.

Labyrinth Training and Consultancy (1994c) *Talking about Vulnerability*. Report of a conference for older people and concerned relatives, friends and neighbours of older people who live alone, for Camden Social Services; Haworth: Labyrinth Training and Consultancy.

Labyrinth Training and Consultancy (1995a) *Evaluation of Ince Community Health Project*, for Ince Community Health Project, Wigan; Haworth: Labyrinth Training and Consultancy.

Labyrinth Training and Consultancy (1995b) *Local Voices: Three Years On*. Workshop Report, Haworth: Labyrinth Training and Consultancy.

Labyrinth Training and Consultancy (1995c) *Moving On*. Report of the National Community Health Conference; Haworth: Labyrinth Training and Consultancy.

Labyrinth Training and Consultancy (1995d) *Review and Development of User and Carer Involvement in Barnsley*, for Barnsley Social Services; Haworth: Labyrinth Training and Consultancy.

Labyrinth Training and Consultancy (1995e) *User and Carer Involvement: Some Examples of Interesting Literature and Practice*, for Barnsley Social Services; Haworth: Labyrinth Training and Consultancy.

Labyrinth Training and Consultancy (1995f) *Greater Chesterton Community Programme: Community Based Needs Assessment*, for North Staffordshire Health Authority and Newcastle-under-Lyme Borough Council; Haworth: Labyrinth Training and Consultancy.

Labyrinth Training and Consultancy (1995g) *Evaluation of the Scottish Community Health Conference, 27–28 March 1995*, for the Health Education Board for Scotland; Haworth: Labyrinth Training and Consultancy.

Labyrinth Training and Consultancy (1995h) *Community Health in Scotland: A Review*, for the Health Education Board for Scotland; Haworth: Labyrinth Training and Consultancy.

Labyrinth Training and Consultancy (1995i) *Tackling Vulnerability Together*. Part II of *Talking About Vulnerability* (Labyrinth 1994c), for Camden Social Services; Haworth: Labyrinth Training and Consultancy.

Labyrinth Training and Consultancy (1996a) *Code of Good Practice for Advocacy in Oldham*, for Oldham Independent Advocacy Steering Group; Haworth: Labyrinth Training and Consultancy.

Labyrinth Training and Consultancy (1996b) *Community Participation in Health Purchasing: A Review of Examples of Interesting Practice*, for Sheffield Health; Haworth: Labyrinth Training and Consultancy.

Labyrinth Training and Consultancy (1996c) *Evaluation and Organisational Review of the Community Psychiatry Research Unit (CPRU)*, for the CPRU, City and Hackney Community NHS Trust; Haworth: Labyrinth Training and Consultancy.

Labyrinth Training and Consultancy (1996d) *Western Isles Health Needs Assessment.* Five Reports, one each for the communities of Barra, Benbecula, Cearns, and South Lochs, and an Overview, for Western Isles Health Board; Haworth: Labyrinth Training and Consultancy.

Labyrinth Training and Consultancy (1996e) *Tunstall Participatory Health Needs Assessment*, for North Staffordshire Health Authority; Haworth: Labyrinth Training and Consultancy.

Labyrinth Training and Consultancy (1996f) *A Brief Overview of Community Development and Health Evaluation Reports within the UK*, for South & West Devon Health Authority and Health Promotion Agency; Haworth: Labyrinth Training and Consultancy.

Labyrinth Training and Consultancy (1996g) *Western Isles Health Needs Assessment: Benbecula Community Survey*, for the Western Isles Health Board; Haworth: Labyrinth Training and Consultancy.

Laughlin, S. and Black, D. (eds) (1995) *Poverty and Health: Tools for Change – Ideas, Analysis, Information, Action*, Birmingham: Public Health Alliance.

Leigh, A. (1988) *Effective Change: Twenty Ways to Make it Happen*, London: Institute of Personnel Management.

Liddington, J. (1984) *The Life and Times of a Respectable Rebel: Selina Cooper 1864–1946*, London: Virago Press.

Llewelyn Davies, M. (ed.) (1977) *Life as we have known it. By Co-operative Working Women*, London: Virago Press.

London Strategic Policy Unit (1986) *Innovation in Everyday Health Care*, Conference on 13–14 February 1986. Conference Papers. London: Greater London Council.

Lovett,, C. (1994) *Advocacy Within Bolton. Report on Advocacy in Bolton: Existing Provision and Developmental Needs*, Bolton: Bolton Advocacy Project, Bolton CVS.

Luck, M. and Jesson, J. (1995) *Community Health Development Evaluation*, Aston Business School.

McNaught, A. (1987) *Health Action and Ethnic Minorities*, Bath: National Community Health Resource (now Community Health UK).

Mansfield CHP (Community Health Project) (1986) *A Report of a Joint Funded Project Between the Health Education Council and Nottinghamshire County Council Social Services Department*, Mansfield Community Health Forum.

Mawhinney, Brian, MP (1994) *Local People Must be Involved in Purchasing*, Press Release (13 April), London.

May, C. and Skinner, S. (1995) *Gaining Ground: Support Pack for Community Groups*, London: Community Development Foundation.

Mayo, M. (1994) *Communities and Caring: The Mixed Economy of Welfare*, New York: St Martin's Press; Basingstoke, Hants.: Macmillan Press.

Medical World/Socialist Health Association (1991) *Health, Wealth and Poverty: Papers on Inequalities in Income and Health*, London: Socialist Health Association.

Merritt, S. (1988), 'Getting it right: monitoring and evaluation in community jobs', *Voluntary Voice Newsletter*, London: London Voluntary Service Council.

Mitchell, M. (1977) *The Hard Way Up: The Autobiography of Hannah Mitchell, Suffragette and Rebel*, London: Virago.

Moody, D. (1992) *Community Participation – A Research Example: Heart Of Our City, Sheffield* (unpublished paper).

Morris, J. (1994) *The Shape of Things to Come? User-Led Social Services*, Social Services Policy Forum, Paper 3, London: National Institute for Social Work.

NCVO (1990) *Effectiveness and the Voluntary Sector: Report of a Working Party*, London: National Council for Voluntary Organisations.

NHS Executive (1994) *Advocacy: A Code of Practice*. Developed by UKAN (United Kingdom Advocacy Network).

NHSME (1992a) *Alliances for Health*, London: Department of Health

NHSME (1992b) *Local Voices: The Views of Local People in Purchasing for Health*, London: Department of Health.

NHSME (1993) *Purchasing for Health – A Framework for Action*, Lancashire: National Health Service Management Executive.

NHSTD (1993a) *Involving Users & Carers in Inter-Agency Management Development*, in 'Developing Managers for Community Care' Series, Bristol: NHS Training Directorate and the Social Services Inspectorate.

NHSTD (1993b) *Managing Services in Partnership: A joint project*, Bristol: NHS Training Directorate and the Social Services Inspectorate.

NHSTD (1994) *Care Management: A Practical Development*, in 'Developing Managers for Community Care' Series, Bristol: NHS Training Directorate and the Social Services Inspectorate.

NIHSS and PHRRC (1992) *Listening to Local Voices: A Guide to Research Methods*, Salford: Nuffield Institute for Health Services Studies and the Public Health Research and Resource Centre.

Ogunsola, A. (1991) 'Representing the Black Community: The Role of Black Community Health Workers', in *'Roots and Branches': Papers from the OU/HEA 1990 Winter School on Community Development and Health*, Milton Keynes: Open University.

Open University (1990) *Baseline Review of Community Development and Health*

Education (CDH), London: Health Education Authority (unpublished document).

Open University (eds) (1991) *'Roots and Branches': Papers from the OU/HEA 1990 Winter School on Community Development and Health*, Milton Keynes: Open University.

Pearse, I. and Crocker, L. (1985) *The Peckham Experiment: A Study of the Living Structure of Society*, Edinburgh: Scottish Academic Press.

Peckham, S., Macdonald, J. and Taylor, P. (1996) *Primary Care and Public Health. Phase I: Project Report*. Report to the Public Health Trust Project Steering Group, Birmingham: Public Health Alliance.

Pedlar, M. and Boutall, J. (1992) *Action Learning for Change: A Resource Book for Managers and Other Professionals*, London: NHS Training Directorate.

Peters, T. (1987) *Thriving on Chaos: A Handbook for a Management Revolution*, London: Macmillan.

PHA (Public Health Alliance) (1989) 'Charter for Public Health', in *Speaking Out for the Public's Health: Papers from a Conference on Public Health Advocacy*, Birmingham: Public Health Alliance.

PHA (Public Health Alliance) (eds) (1992) *Community Development and Health: Reclaiming the National Agenda*. Report of a National Seminar, 22–23 May 1991, Birmingham: Public Health Alliance.

Plant, R. (1987) *Managing Change and Making it Stick*, London: Fontana.

Powell, M. (1992) *Healthy Alliances: A Report to the Conference on Healthgain*, London: King's Fund.

Prout, A. and Deverell, K. (1995) *Working With Diversity: Building Communities. Evaluating the MESMAC Project*. London: Health Education Authority.

Rawson, M. and Macredie, S. (undated) *How's Everything Going? Impact 3 Community Health Project*. Evaluation Protocol.

Rawson, M. and Macredie, S. (1996) *How's Everything Going? Impact 3 Community Health Project*. Evaluation Year 2 Review.

Reason, L. (1985) *Catford Community Health Project: Evaluation Project*, London: CCHP.

Ritchie, C. (1992) *Heeley Health Project: Evaluation of Activities, April 1990 – July 1991*, Community Operational Research Unit (CORU), Northern College, Barnsley.

Salt, C., Schweitzer, P and Wilson, M. (eds) (1983) *Of Whole Heart Cometh Hope: Centenary Memories of the Co-operative Women's Guild*, London: Age Exchange Theatre Company, Greater London Council.

SCCD, UKACW and FCWTG (1995) 'Organisational Viewpoints' in *Community Development Journal*, 30(2).

Scottish Office (1992) *Scotland's Health: A Challenge to Us All*. A Policy Statement. London: HMSO.

Scott-Samuel, A. (1997) *The Jakarta Declaration on Health Promotion into the 21st Century*. A Summary. Department of Health, Liverpool University.

Sheffield District Health Authority (1988) 'Heart Of Our City' (unpublished funding application).

Skinner, S. (1997) *Building Community Strengths: A Resource Book on Capacity Building*, London: Community Development Foundation.

Smith, C. (1982) *Community Based Health Initiatives: A Handbook for Voluntary Groups*, Bath: Community Health UK.

Smithies, J. (1991) 'Management theory and community development theory', in *'Roots and Branches': Papers from the OU/HEA 1990 Winter School on Community Development and Health*, Milton Keynes: Open University.

Smithies, J. (1992) 'The New Role of Health Authorities: Involving Local Care' in *The Public as Partners: A Tool-Box for Involving Local People in Commissioning Health Care*, Cambridge: Healthgain Conference.

Smithies, J. and Adams, L. (1990) *Community Participation in Health Promotion*, London: Health Education Authority.

Spray, J. (1992) 'Health Education Authority', in Public Health Alliance (eds) (1992), *Community Development and Health: Reclaiming the National Agenda*. Report of a National Seminar, 22–23 May 1991, Birmingham: Public Health Alliance.

SSI (1995) *Community Care Monitoring*, Social Services Inspectorate (North of England Region), Department of Health.

Thamesdown Evaluation Project (1994) *Enhancing Practice through Evaluation: Opportunities for the Voluntary Sector*. A review of the Thamesdown Evaluation Project.

Thunhurst, C. and Postma, S. (1989) *The Health Profile of the City of Stoke-on-Trent*, Leeds: Nuffield Institute for Health Service Studies.

Townsend, P., Whitehead, M. and Davidson, N. (eds) (1992) *Inequalities in Health*, Harmondsworth: Penguin.

UKHFAN *UK Health For All Network Newsletter* Liverpool: UKHFAN Ltd.

UKHFAN (UK Health For All Network) (1991) *Community Participation for Health For All*, Community Participation Group; Liverpool: UK Health For All Network.

Watt, A. (1986) *Community Health Initiatives: Clarifying the Complexities within the Community Health Movement*, Papers from the conference 'Community Development in Health: Addressing the Confusions', London: King's Fund Centre.

Watters, M. (1995) *Towards a Strategy for Carers: Multi-Agency Research on Carers in Tameside*, West Pennine Resource Centre and the Policy Unit, Tameside Metropolitan Borough Council.

Webster, C. (1992) 'Inequalities in Health: The Failure of the NHS in Post-war Britain', in *Health, Wealth and Poverty: Papers on Inequalities in Income and Health*, London: Socialist Health Association.

Webster, C. (1993) 'Health Advocacy in History', in *Speaking Out for the Public's Health: Papers from a Conference on Public Health Advocacy*, Birmingham: Public Health Alliance.

Webster, G. (1989) *Community Development and Health Promotion: Links Between Theory and Practice*, unpublished paper.

Webster, G, (1992) 'Setting the Scene', in Public Health Alliance (eds) (1992), *Community Development and Health: Reclaiming the National Agenda*. Report of a National Seminar, 22–23 May 1991, Birmingham: Public Health Alliance.

Whitehead, M. (1992) 'The Social Determinants of Ill Health', in *Health, Wealth and Poverty: Papers on Inequalities in Income and Health*, London: Socialist Health Association.

Wilcox, D. (1994) The *Guide to Effective Participation*, Brighton: Partnership Books.

Wilkinson, R.G. (1992) 'Income and Health', in *Health, Wealth and Poverty: Papers on Inequalities in Income and Health*, London: Socialist Health Association.

World Commission on Environment and Development (1987) *Our Common Future: From One Earth to One World*, New York: Oxford University Press.

World Health Organization (1985) Targets for Health For All: Targets in Support of the European Strategy for Health For All, WHO Regional Office for Europe.

World Health Organization (1986), 'The Ottawa Charter', Geneva: World Health Organisation.

World Health Organization (1988) 'Creating Healthy Public Policy', quoted in 'Adelaide recommendations: Healthy Public Policy', *Health Promotion* 3(2): 183–186.

Index

(n.b. Page references for boxes, figures and tables are shown in *italic*.)

Foxdenton School for children with
  special needs 107–8
Freeman, R. 36
French, W.L. 218 n.1
Funnell, R. 42

*Gaining Ground: Support Pack for
  Community Groups* (May and
  Skinner) 209
Gamble, D.N. 87
General Board of Health 10
General Household Survey 276
general practitioners (GPs) 255–6, 259,
  273, 275, 276, 280
  fundholders 36, 75, 141, 152, 259
Glasgow 12
  community health projects in 133, 156
  participatory health needs assess-
    ment in 156
governance 51
Government Urban Aid Programme 7
Granton Community Health Project
  132, 133
Greater Chesterton Community Health
  Project 129, 284
Greater London Council 18, *32*
Green, J. 15, 187–90
Guide to Community Health Projects
  (CHIRU/LCHR) 20–1, 131

Hackney, London 238
Hancock, Trevor 58 n.2,n.3
Hanmer, J. 6, 9, 10
Harlow, Essex
  National Women's Health Conference
    held in 21
Harris, R.T. 213
health, definition of 60, 131, 186
Health Action Areas 159
Health Action Zones (HAZ) 44, 49
health authorities
  and advocacy 105, 110, 116, 280–1
  and community health projects 129,
    141–2, *149*
  community participation strategies of
    252, 253–7, 258–9
    involving service users and carers
      273, 275, 280–1
  culture of 38, 231, 255
  funding and resourcing of 204, 234

and health needs assessment *see*
  health needs assessment, participatory
role of 36, 37, 39, 43, 50, 54, 65, 96,
  104, 152
see also health purchasing; *and under
  names of individual health authorities*, e.g. Airedale Health Authority
health centres 136–7, 197, 275
Health Education Authority (HEA) 52,
  70, 171, 178, 182
  Professional and Community Devel-
    opment Division (PCD) 21–30
    passim, 33
  budget of 24–5, 27, 28, 30, *33*
  'Roots and Branches Winter School'
    of 27, *33*
  see also Health Education Council
    (HEC)
Health Education Board for Scotland
  (HEBS) 31, *34*, 285
Health Education Council (HEC) 23, 24,
  70
  see also Health Education Authority
    (HEA)
'Health For All by the Year 2000' (World
  Health Organization) 5, 11–13, 15,
  37, 41, 49, 51, 69–70, 90, 171, 172,
  213, *230*, 244, 258, 281
  aims of 11, 46, 68
Health Improvement Programmes 43–4,
  68
health needs assessment, participatory
  Ch.9, 224, 257
  changing approach to 37, 98, 151–2
  checklist for obtaining local involve-
    ment 154–5, *155*
  context of 152–4
  'five elements' model used in 237,
    238, 244–7
  methodology used in 37–8, 154–5,
    156–7, 161, 162
  in North Yorkshire 227
  in Oldham 156–7, 163
  organisation development and 38,
    164–7, 202, 227
  requirements for 154, 166–7
  selecting a geographical area 158–64
    definition of a community and 164

United States
  citizen advocacy movement in 104
  community development work in
    206–7
Urban Aid 72
*User and Carer Involvement: Some
  Examples of Interesting Literature and
  Practice* (Labyrinth) 104
user forums 105, 122, 267
user groups 10, 14, 15, 36, 50, 54–5, 62,
  69, *83*, 84, 99, 100, 104, 105, 108,
  116, 117, 262, 264, 265, 270, 271, 273
user-led social services, model of 125

Validity and the Research Process
  (Brinberg and McGrath) 170
validity of research 170–2, 180
Voluntary Action Manchester 272
Voluntary and Community Division 53
voluntary sector 44, 46, 66, 135, 136,
  206, 223
  and community care 104, 272–3, 280–1
  Council for Voluntary Services 74, 118
  funding for 52–3, 139, 258
  identifying training needs for 233
  Joint Consultative Committee (JCC)
    268
  National Council for Voluntary
    Organisations (NCVO) 14, 19–20,
    32, 52, 53, 285
  new role of 52–3
  organisation development within 123
  partnerships with 42, 43, 45, 48, 50,
    53, 159, 203
Voluntary Services Unit 53
Voluntary Voice 172

Wales
  community development and health
    in 31, *34*, 238, 279–80
  national strategy for health in 31, 36,
    44
Watt, A. 14
Watters, M. 275–7
WCCUIN *see* Wiltshire Community
  Care User Involvement Network
  (WCCUIN)
Webster, C. 11, 47
Webster, G. 12, 28
Weil, M.O. 87
Welfare State

benefits 204, 274
establishment of 6
Wells Park Health Project, Sydenham
  18, 136–7, 286
West Bowling Community Health
  Action Project 130, 131, 286
West Lancashire
  carers' needs in 273–5
West Yorkshire Community Health
  Training Project 92
Western Isles
  participatory health needs assess-
    ment in 165–7, 202
Western Isles Health Board 165
Whitehead, M. 11, 47
WHRRIC *see* Women's Health and
  Reproductive Rights Information
  Centre (WHRRIC)
Wigan
  Ince Community Health Project in
    72–4, 185–6
Wigan and Bolton Health Authority 72
Wilcox, D. 84
Wilkinson, R.G. 47
Wiltshire Community Care Consulta-
  tion Conference (1991) 271
Wiltshire Community Care User
  Involvement Network (WCCUIN)
  268, 271–2, 286
  areas of involvement 271
  funding of 272
  organisational infrastructure of 271
Wiltshire Health Authority 271
Women's Aid Groups 14–15
Women's Health and Reproductive
  Rights Information Centre
  (WHRRIC) 10, 21
Women's Health Conference (Liver-
  pool, 1989) 26
women's health initiatives 8, 9–10, 14–
  15, 18, 21, 24, 25, 26, 27, 29, 32, 33,
  83, 92, 131, 132, 198, 209
  see also equal opportunities policies
Women's Peace Movement 14
World Commission on Environment
  and Development 55, 87
World Health Organisation 5, 11, 12, 26,
  51, 68, 69–70, 131
  Constitution of 60

Youth Action Project 142